Application of Newer Forms of Therapeutic Energy in Urology

Provided as a service to urology by

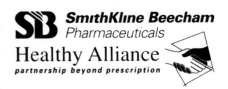

SmithKline Beecham
Pharmaceuticals

Healthy Alliance
partnership beyond prescription

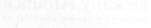

Application of Newer Forms of Therapeutic Energy in Urology

Edited by

Michael Marberger

Professor and Chairman,
Department of Urology,
University of Vienna, Austria

I S I S
MEDICAL
M E D I A

—

Oxford

© 1995 by Isis Medical Media Ltd
Saxon Beck, 58 St Aldates
Oxford, OX1 1ST, UK

First published 1995

British Library Cataloguing in Publication Data. A catalogue record for this title is available from the British Library

ISBN 1 899066 12 8

Marberger (Michael)
Application of Newer Forms of Therapeutic Energy in Urology Michael Marberger

Always refer to the manufacturer's Prescribing Information before prescribing drugs cited in this book.

Set by
Marksbury Typesetting Ltd, Midsomer Norton, Bath, UK

Printed by
Dah Hua Printing Press Co. Ltd, Hong Kong

Distributed by
Times Mirror International Publishers, Customer Service Centre, Unit 1, 3 Sheldon Way, Larkfield, Aylesford, Kent, ME20 6SF, UK

Contents

CONTENTS

List of Contributors

Clément-Claude Abbou MD
Chairman, Service d'Urologie, Hôpital Henri Mondor, 51 avenue du Marechal de Lattre, 94010 Crétei, France

Laurent Boccon-Gibod MD
Professor, Service d'Urologie, Hôpital Saint Louis, 1 avenue Claude Vellefaux, 75475 Paris, Cedex 19, France

Daniel Beurton MD
Service d'Urologie, Hopital Ambroise Paré, 9 Avenue Charles de Gaulle, F-92104 Boulogne, France

Jacques Biserte MD
Professeur des Universités, Praticien Hospitalie, Services d'Urologie, C.H.U. Lille, Place de Verdun, F-59037, Lille, France

Francis Callot MD
Bruker's company consultant, Société Bruker, Wissembourg, France

Françoise Carpentier MD
Praticien Hospitalier, Senor Résident, Hopital Victor Provo, Service Anatomo-Pathologique, 17 Boulevard L'acordaire, Service Urologie, BP 359-59056, Roubaix, France

Jean Y. Chapelon PhD
Senior Bioscientist, Inserm U 281, 151 cours A. Thomas, 69003, Lyon, France

Maurice Chive
Professeur des Universités–Faculté des Sciences, I.E.M.N. CHS UMR. 9929 CNRS, Université des Sciences et Technologie de Lille, Bat P4, 59655, Villeneuve D'Ascq, Lille II, France

Yong-Hyun Cho   MD, Dr. Med. Sc.
Associate Professor, Department of Urology, St. Mary's Hospital, Catholic University Medical College, #62 Yoidodong, Yongdungpoku, 150-010, Seoul, Korea

Pierre Colombeau   MD
Professor and Chairman, Department of Urology, C.H.U. Dupuytren, 2 Av. Alexis Carrel, 87942 Limoges, France

Anthony J. Costello   FRACS, MB BS
Head, Department of Urology, St. Vincent's Hospital, Victoria Parade, Fitzroy, Melbourne, Australia

Robert S. Cowles III   MD FACS
Clinical Assistant Professor of Surgery, Emory University, 3193 Howell Mill Road NW, Suite 229, Atlanta, Ga. 30327, USA

Jean J.M.C.H de la Rosette   MD, PhD
Director of Centre of Prostatic Disease, Department of Urology, University Hospital, Nijmejen, P.O. Box 9101, 6500 HB, Nijmegen, The Netherlands

Dimitri Demetriou   MD
Chef de Clinique Assistant, Hopital Victor Provo, Boulevard Lacordaire F-59100 Roubaix, France

Marian Devonec   MD, PhD
Urology Department, Antiquaille Hospital, Lyon 69321, France

Jacques Fermanian
Département de Biostatistiques, Hôpital Necker, Paris, France

Albert Gelet   MD
Associate Chief of Urology and Transplantation Department, Eduard Herriot Hospital, 69 437 Lyon, Cedex 03, France

Benad Goldwasser   MD
Chairman, Department of Urology, The Sheba Medical Center, Tel-Hashomer 52621, Israel

Bertrand Guillonneau   MD
Urological Surgeon, Department of Urology, C.M.C. de la Porte de Choisy, F-75013 Paris, France

Fadi Habib   MD
*The Division of Urology, The Toronto Hospital, 200 Elizabeth Street,
Toronto, Ontario, M5G 2C4, Canada*

David Hald
*Department of Urology, Miller Children's Hospital, Long Beach
Memorial Medical Center, University of California, Irvine, California,
USA*

Mohamed Harouni   MD
*Urological Surgeon, Department of Urology, C.M.C. de la Porte de
Choisy, F-75013 Paris, France*

Bagdad Hattab
*Assistant generaliste and Resident, Hopital Victor Provo, Service
Urologie, 17 Boulevard L'accordaire, BP 359-59056, Roubaix, France*

Stefan Hessel   DR. ENG
*Professor, Department of Electrical Engineering, Munich University,
Munich, Germany*

Eiji Higashihara   MD
*Professor and Chairman, Department of Urology, School of Medicine,
Kyorin University, 6-20-2 Shinkawa, Mitaka, Tokyo 181, Japan*

Klaus Höfner
*Department of Urology, Hannover Medical School, Konstanty-
Gutschow Strasse 8, 30625, Hannover, Germany*

Alfons Hofstetter   MD
*Professor and Chairman, Department of Urology, Munich University,
Marchionistrasse 15, D-81377, Munich, Germany*

Patrice Houdelette   MD
*Professor and Chairman, Urology Department, Val de Grace Hospital,
F-75014 Paris, France*

Guntram Hubmann   MD
Department of Urology, D 67434 Neustadt/Weinstrasse, Germany

Alain Jardin
9 Boulevard du Temple, 75003 Paris, France

Udo Jonas DR
Professor and Chairman, Department of Urology, Hannover Medical School, Konstanty-Gutschow Strasse, 8-30625 Hannover, Germany

John N. Kabalin MD
Assistant Professor of Urology, Stanford University School of Medicine; Chief, Urology, Urology (112C), Palo Alto V.A. Medical Center, 3801 Miranda Avenue, Palo Alto, California, 94304, USA

Jenz Kemper MD
Department of Urology, D 12205 Berlin, Germany

Anthony Khim
Department of Urology, Miller Children's Hospital, Long Beach Memorial Medical Center, University of California, Irvine, California, USA

Jin Ho Kim
Department of Urology, St. Mary's Hospital, Catholic University Medical College, #62 Yoidodong, Yongdungpoku, 150–010, Seoul, Korea

Sae Woong Kim
Department of Urology, St. Mary's Hospital, Catholic University Medical College, #62 Yoidodong, Yongdungpoku, 150–010, Seoul, Korea

Helmut Krah
Department of Urology, Hannover Medical School, Konstanty-Gutschow Strasse, 8-30625, Hannover, Germany

Markus Kuczyk
Department of Urology, Hannover Medical School, Konstanty-Gutschow Strasse, 8-30625, Hannover, Germany

Alain Le Duc
Professor and Chairman, Department of Urology, Hopital Saint-Louis, 1 avenue Claude Vellefaux, 75475 Paris, Cedex 19, France

Stephan Madersbacher MD
Department of Urology, University of Vienna, Währinger Gürtel 18-20, A-1090 Vienna, Austria

Michael Marberger   MD
Professor and Chairman, Department of Urology, University of Vienna,
Währinger Gürtel 18-20, A-1090 Vienna, Austria

Wilfried Martin
Department of Urology, Ruhr University of Bochum, Marienhospital,
Widumer Strasse 8, D-44627, Herne, Germany

Brigitte Mauroy   PU-PH
Professeur des Universités, Practicien Hospitalier, Service Universitaire
d'Urologie, CH Roubaix, France

Etienne Mazeman   MD
Professeur des Universités, Practicien Hospitalier, Chef de Service,
Clinique Urologique, CHU Lille, France

Philippe Menguy   MD
Ambroise Paré Hospital, F-13006 Marseille, France

Stephan Mölhoff   MD
Department of Urology, Üniversität Klinikum Essen, D-45147 Essen,
Germany

Rolf Muschter   MD
Department of Urology, Grosshadem Clinic, Munich University,
Marchioninistrasse 15, D-81377, Munich, Germany

Christine Payan
Comité d'Evaluation et de Diffusion des Innovations Technologiques,
Paris, France

Michel Peneau   MD
Department of Urology, CHR Orléans, 45032 Orléans, France

Aaron P. Perlmutter   MD, PhD
Director, Brady Prostate Center; Assistant Professor of Urology,
Department of Urology, James Buchanan Brady Foundation, New York
Hospital - Cornell Medical Center, 525 E 68th Street, New York, NY
10021, USA

Paul Perrin   MD
Professor and Chairman, Department of Urology, Hopital de
L'Antiquaille, 1 rue de l'Antiquaille, F-69321 Lyon, Cedex 05, France

Hans Rall MD
Department of Urology, D-90491, Nürnberg 20, Germany

Jacob Ramon MD
Consultant Urologist, The Chaim Sheba Medical Center, Tel-Hashomer 52621, Israel

François Richard
Service d'Urologie, Hôpital Pitié-Salpétrière, Paris, France

Theodor Senge MD
Professor and Chairman, Department of Urology, Ruhr University of Bochum, Marienhospital, Widumer Strasse 8, D-44627 Herne, Germany

Claude C. Schulman
Professor of Urology and Chief, Department of Urology, University Clinics of Brussels, Erasme Hospital, 808 route de Lennik, B-1070 Brussels, Belgium

Harald Schulze MD, PD
Department of Urology, Ruhr University of Bochum, Marienhospital, Widumer Strasse 8, D-44627, Herne, Germany

Allan M. Shanberg MD, FACS, FAAP
Clinical Professor of Surgery-Urology, University of California - Irvine, Director, Reider Laser Center, Long Beach Memorial Medical Center, 2865 Atlantic Avenue, Suite 217, Long Beach, California, 90806, USA

Jeani Pierre Sozanski
Ingénieur de Recherche, U.279 I.N.S.E.R.M., 13/17 rue du Professeur Calmette, 59000, Lille, France

Hong Kie Tan
Department of Urology, Hannover Medical School, Konstanty-Gutschow Strasse, 8-30625, Hannover, Germany

Ants Toi
The Department of Radiologic Sciences, The Toronto Hospital, 200 Elizabeth, Street, Toronto, Ontario, M5G 2C4, Canada

John Trachtenberg MD, FRCS (C), FACS
Professor, The Division of Urology, The Toronto Hospital, 200 Elizabeth Street, Toronto, Ontario, M5G 2C4, Canada

Mutsumi Uchida MD
*Department of Urology, Kyoto Prefectural University of Medicine,
Kawaramachi-Hirokoji, Kyoto 602, Japan*

Guy Vallancien MD
*Professor of Urology, Department of Urology, C.M.C. de la Porte de
Choisy, F-75013 Paris, France*

Bruno Veillon MD
*Urological Surgeon, Department of Urology, C.M.C. de la Porte de
Choisy, F-75013 Paris, France*

Catherine Viens-Bitker
*Comité d'Evaluation et de Diffusion des Innovations Technologiques,
Paris, France*

Andrew C. von Eschenbach MD
*Department of Urology, The University of Texas, M.D. Anderson
Cancer Center, 1515 Holcombe Boulevard, Houston, Texas, 77030,
USA*

Hiroki Watanabe MD
*Department of Urology, Kyoto Prefectural University of Medicine,
Kawaramachi-Hirokoji, Kyoto 602, Japan*

Eugene Yeung MD
*The Department of Radiologic Sciences, The Toronto Hospital, 200
Elizabeth Street, Toronto, Ontario, M5G 2C4, Canada*

Kimihiko Yoneda MD
*Department of Urology, Kyoto Prefectural University of Medicine,
Kawaramachi-Hirokoji, Kyoto 602, Japan*

Moon Soo Yoon MD
*Professor of Urology, Department of Urology, St. Mary's Hospital,
Catholic University Medical College, #62 Yoidodong, Yongdungpoku,
150-010, Seoul, Korea*

Alexandre R. Zlotta MD
*Department of Urology, University Clinics of Brussels, Erasme Hospital,
808 route de Lennik, B-1070 Brussels, Belgium*

Preface

It is not only fine feathers that make fine birds
Aesop, 550 BC

It is an old dream in medicine to cut, destroy or ablate diseased tissue within the body without damage to surrounding structures. Modern radiotherapy has achieved much towards this goal, but the ratio between reliable tissue destruction in the target zone and toxicity to intervening tissues is still far from satisfactory. Advanced endoscopic and imaging techniques today permit the access of energy deep into the body without the need for mutilating surgery. Traditional mechanical and electrosurgical cutting can be utilized in this manner, but recent developments in laser, ultrasound, microwave and radiofrequency technology seem to offer substantial advantages. Percutaneous application of therapeutic energy without the need of direct manipulation of the patient appears even more attractive. The success story of extracorporeal shock wave lithotripsy has shown the way—newer forms of energy hitherto poorly understood can, indeed, be utilized for defined minimally invasive surgical action.

In our era of confidence in technological progress, almost any effect can be achieved with the wide range of modern technology currently available. The problem lies in the need for clinical practicability. The true value of a new therapeutic approach depends on the correct balance between technical complexity, morbidity, efficacy and cost, with clear advantages over the standard treatment. This is not a fixed relation; a significant reduction of morbidity, such as by the avoidance of anaesthesia, may counterbalance a lesser degree of efficacy compared with the conventional treatment. Cost is a factor highly dependent on the health care system: the cost of disposable materials may be prohibitive in some parts of the world and acceptable in others. Moreover, technical development is an ongoing process, and apparently minor improvements may suddenly result in a clinical breakthrough.

Unbiased clinical evaluation can hardly be expected from the innovator. Apart from an understandable inclination towards the favourable aspects of his development, technical details may give him tunnel vision, so that he cannot see the wood for the trees. Other clinicians frequently lack the technical knowledge to comprehend the innovation and tend to favour the conventional approach with which they are familiar. The situation is further complicated by the attention this field receives in the lay news media. Incompletely informed, frequently by the medical authorities promoting a new technology, the lay public exerts 'market forces' that render fair clinical evaluation almost impossible. If the field is not to be left entirely to government regulations, the medical profession has to provide appropriate guidelines for the evaluation process, and publications giving objective information.

Urologists are traditionally to the fore in utilizing newer forms of therapeutic energy in clinical practice. Specifically, benign and malignant diseases of the prostate may be the first clinical entities where patients may actually profit from these advances. Realizing this, the Sociètè Internationale d'Urologie designated a monograph on this topic. Newer approaches in the use of microwaves, radiofrequency waves, ultrasound energy and lasers were to be covered. A previous monograph was related to alternative treatment modalities of urinary stones. Stone-related methods are, therefore, excluded from this volume, but the use of mechanical energy for non-urolithiasis indications is contained here. Although not new, discussion of cryosurgical techniques has been added for reasons of actuality. Recent developments in electrosurgery may have future implications in urology, but at present they still appear too speculative for a detailed discussion.

In the traditional SIU format, the main aspects of the topic are presented in unprejudiced overviews, which are supplemented by articles on specific techniques by the leading pioneers in the field. Readers can draw their own conclusions.

Michael Marberger
April 1995

Mechanical energy in urology for non-lithiasis treatment

1

E. Higashihara

Introduction

This chapter reviews those forms of mechanical energy used in urology, other than those used for urolithiasis treatment.

Energy is defined as the ability of one system to empower another system. It is classified by the form of accumulation or transfer, such as mechanical energy, thermal energy, chemical energy and nuclear energy. Energy can change from one form to another. During energy conversion, energy is conserved for all isolated mechanical systems. The dynamic energy field is also called mechanical energy or external energy. Mechanical energy consists of kinetic energy and potential energy.

The types of mechanical energy reviewed in this chapter include ultrasonic ballistic energy, water energy and shock wave energy used for non-lithiasis treatment. A historical perspective is beyond the scope of this chapter; however, the use of ultrasonic ballistic energy has a long history and many excellent reports and reviews are available.[1-3]

The water jet scalpel is a relatively new instrument of which there is, as yet, insufficient experience in the urological field. In this regard, this review may help readers to develop an understanding of the potential of this tool.

Shock wave treatment for tumours is now in the experimental phase. Clinical application must await conclusive proof that shock waves do not enhance tumour metastasis.

Water energy: water jet scalpel

General considerations

Water energy can be used as a water jet scalpel, created by jetting water through a small nozzle under high pressure. Water jet energy is used in civil engineering, for example in soil improvement in reclaimed land, renovation of general industrial facilities, excavation or jet piling. Even iron or steel can be cut easily with an abrasive water jet, using solid particles in suspension. Nuclear power plant facilities can be dismantled using an abrasive water jet system combined with a remote control and collection system for radioactive waste.

In Fig. 1.1, the relation between the distance from the nozzle outlet and the falling curve of the pressure is compared for water and/or air jets. In medical applications of the water jet, the handpiece is usually held within 5 cm of the target tissue and no decrease in the pressure is anticipated. The cutting mechanism is hydrostatic pressure enhanced by mixing abrasives such as iron filings or other solid powders with the water (abrasive water jet). Water jets can separate structures depending on the intensity of the water jet pressure. Conversely, when appropriate pressure and nozzle size are chosen, the water jet selectively cuts certain materials while leaving others undamaged. The pressures used for different purposes are shown in Fig. 1.2.

Medical applications

For medical use, a pressure between 10 and 50 kg/cm^2 is selected. A water jet dissector has been developed for hepatectomy.[4,5] Surgery time and perioperative blood loss were reduced compared with those associated with the use of an ultrasonic surgical aspirator.[6,7] The water jet scalpel removes only parenchymatous tissue, using the impact energy of the water jet. The blood vessels, nerves and bile ducts are left undamaged. In addition, as the water impinges on the vascular structures and flows around them, it can eliminate tissue located behind the vessels. This unique characteristic in dissection results in tissue skeletonization and facilitates haemostasis by electrocautery or suturing. The size of blood vessels that remain undamaged using a water jet scalpel is approximately 200 μm, whereas that when using an ultrasonic surgical aspirator is approximately 500 μm; thus, there is preservation of thinner blood vessels and less blood

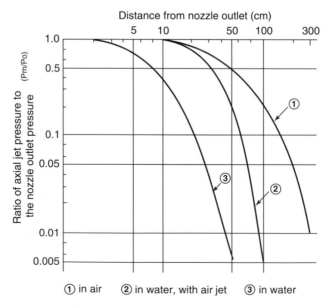

Fig. 1.1. Relation between distance from the nozzle outlet and the decreasing pressure of a water jet in air (curve 1), in water, with an air jet (curve 2) and in water (curve 3). (Reproduced from ref. 58 with permission.)

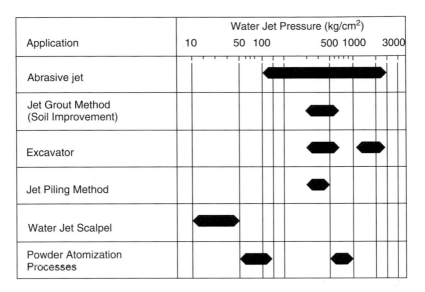

Fig. 1.2. Water jet pressures used for different purposes. (Reproduced from ref. 58 with permission.)

loss when using the water jet scalpel than when using the ultrasonic aspirator. The water jet also cleans the area by irrigation, washing blood and fragmented tissue away from the surgical field, while debris and fluids are collected simultaneously by a suction pump.

The water jet dissector (Aqua Jet Mes) developed by Sugino Machine Limited (Toyama, Japan) consists of a 100 g handpiece connected to a control console by a flexible tube. The inner diameter of the handpiece nozzle is 150 μm. The pressure can be adjusted from 0 to 20 kg/cm^2, depending on the tissue being treated, and water flow varies from 0 to 43 ml/min, according to the pressure selected. Usually, physiological saline is used instead of water. The handpiece incorporates an on–off switch, and the water jet nozzle is covered by a transparent hollow tip through which irrigated saline, blood and tissue fragments are aspirated.

In urology, partial nephrectomy, nephrolithotomy, and nerve-sparing surgery in prostatectomy and in retroperitoneal lymph node dissection, are all indications for use of the water jet scalpel.

Shock wave energy for non-lithiasis treatment

Side effects of extracorporeal shock wave lithotripsy (ESWL), such as haematuria, tissue injury and transient decrease in renal function, have been encountered in many cases.[8,9] Investigation into the causes of such side effects has disclosed the mechanisms of tissue injury and has led to the application of shock wave energy for tumoricidal purposes.

Experiments to delineate the effects of shock wave energy on malignant tumours are of three types: first is basic research on the mechanisms that generate cavitation and cavitation-related cytocidal effects;[10] second is research in vitro, investigating the effects of shock waves on cultured cell lines with or without a combination of cytotoxic drugs or cytokines; third is research in vivo, using tumours implanted in animals. The results obtained in the systems in vitro are not applicable to the systems in vivo because of the different underlying mechanisms causing the cytotoxic effects of shock waves in the two systems. As the crucially important issue concerning the possibility of enhanced metastasis of malignant cells following shock wave application has not been satisfactorily resolved, clinical application should await clarification.

Physical aspects and basic research

Weak acoustic shock waves, which are used for the clinical treatment of lithiasis, are a novel source of mechanical energy. No significant thermal effects are induced by focused shock waves, and their biological effects are mainly purely mechanical interactions and transient cavitation processes.[11,12]

Cavitation phenomenon

If a negative pressure greater than the ambient pressure exists in a liquid, then the liquid may fail under the stress.[13] The focused shock wave consists of both positive and negative pressures up to 114 and 10 MPa, respectively, and this negative pressure is sufficient to cause cavitation.[14] Shock waves produce liquid failure at numerous discrete sites near the focus. When the liquid fails, the vapour-filled cavities that are initially developed ultimately collapse with enormous force.[15] Cavitation bubbles appear when the liquid pressure rapidly decreases below the liquid vapour pressure. Cavitation can be described as boiling at an ambient temperature.[10]

Williams et al[16] observed shock wave-induced cavitation using a resonant bubble detector, which can detect bubbles from 3 to 5 μm in diameter. They detected bubbles resulting from shock wave-induced cavitation in water and blood in vitro, but could not observe cavitation occurring within the intact vascular systems of dogs in vivo.[16] They attributed this to the fact that, in vivo, blood is thoroughly filtered, cleaned and purified by various active and passive processes, and it simply may not contain any nuclei suitable for bubble production. Although their experiments did not preclude cavitation occurring in tissues or bubbles with a diameter other than 3–5 μm, that cavitation may actually occur in vivo is far from certain. Using an ultrasonic imaging system, Kuwahara suggested that the hyperechoic region at the focal area in the dog kidney was evidence of cavitation in vivo.[10] Conclusive evidence of the cavitation phenomenon in living tissue has not yet been provided and awaits further study.

Liquid microjets

Acoustic cavitation causes severe erosion in materials exposed to cavitation fields.[15,17] This erosion is due to cavitation-induced microjets. During the collapse of cavitation bubbles, high-speed liquid microjets are created. When the interface of a collapsing bubble is unstable, any small disturbance near the bubble initiates bubble deformation. This deformity results in the bubble plunging into the microjets on one side and leads to a funnel-shape protrusion on the other side of the bubble wall.[18] Microjet velocities are expected to range from 130 to 170 m/s, and it is accepted that high-speed microjets are the primary mechanism of mechanical force in stone disintegration.[15] These microjets are also considered to be the cause of undesirable side effects in tissues in systems in vitro and in vivo.

High temperature

The high speed of the breakdown of the bubble causes adiabatic compression of gas inside the bubble without heat exchange with the surrounding medium; adiabatic compression results in a local temperature increase. The temperature and pressure within a collapsing cavity have been calculated to reach levels of 10 000 K and 1000 MPa (10 000 kg/cm^2), respectively.[15] Theoretically, a high temperature is expected even with a modest negative pressure.[18] Direct measurement of cavitation temperature using sonoluminescence spectra in silicon oil has demonstrated an effective cavitation temperature of 5075 ± 156 K, which was lower than the predicted value.[19] This cavitation-related rise in the temperature was measured in vitro or calculated on the basis of many assumptions, and is therefore valid only under certain circumstances.

Solving the equation of thermal conductivity, Filipczynski et al[20] estimated the temperature rise in vivo to be less than 1°C during lithotripsy of 3000 shock waves at a repetition rate of 1 or 2 Hz. The temperature rise in the second focus area during a single shock wave was estimated to be roughly 10^{-2}°C, supposing a waterlike medium with an absorption coefficient of 0.1 Np/cm and the absence of heat transfer to the surrounding medium.[11,21] The actual temperature elevation might be even less, owing to tissue attenuation and the cooling effect of blood circulation.

Free radicals

Inside a collapsing bubble, the pressure and temperature generated can induce homolytic cleavage of the molecule and lead to the formation of free radicals,[10] which are anticipated to be tumoricidal.

It has been shown that free radicals are generated in a cell-free medium[22,23] as well as in a suspended cell solution in the focal area of shock waves.[22] Morgan et al[23] have demonstrated that the shock waves generate free radicals and this effect is increased by the acoustic interface. Suhr et al[22] have shown that scavengers of free radicals increase the survival rate of the L1210 mouse leukaemia cell line treated by shock waves, In addition, inhibitors of the defence enzymes superoxide dismutase and catalase reduce the survival rate of the suspended cell line after exposure to shock waves.[22] However, in systems in vivo it is not clear to what extent the cavitation-related free radicals contribute to the shock wave-induced cytotoxicity. One thousand shock waves induce the same free-radical oxidation as 1100 rad cobalt-60 gamma ionizing irradiation.[23] Whereas 1100 rad cobalt irradiation produces marked cell damage, little effect is noted on exposure to 1000 shock waves. In systems in vivo, cavitation and/or cavitation-related free-radical generation may be either absent or attenuated.[23] Mechanical forces probably have an important role in tumoricidal effects of shock waves in systems in vivo, whereas cavitation-induced free radicals in addition to mechanical energy contribute to the cytotoxic effects in models in vitro.

Liquid flow

When shock waves are propagated in air, they also induce a flow velocity that races behind the shock wave front. The flow velocity, termed 'blast', acts as a primary force in destroying materials. Liquid flow is much less in water than in air because of the limited compressibility of water.[10] Nevertheless, as long as liquid flow exists behind an underwater shock wave it may act as a shearing force, because it propagates in a direction radiating from the axis of shock wave propagation.

Compression and tensile stress

In addition to microjets,[15] compression and tensile stress play an important part in disintegrating stones.[24,25] These forces may act when there is a difference in acoustic impedance between the tissues and organs. However, there is no information about the role of these forces in tissue injury.

Experiments in vitro

Effects of shock waves

Since Russo et al[26] showed that electrohydraulically generated shock waves can be cytotoxic to tumour cells in vivo and in vitro, many similar results have been reported.[26–30] Apart from immediately lethal effects (such as fragmentation of cells), permeabilization of the plasma membrane, mitochondrial swelling, altered vimentin structure, cytotoxic cisternae and nuclear changes have been described.[27–29] Shock wave-induced cytotoxicity has been demonstrated using not only an electrohydraulic (hydroelectric) but also an electromagnetic or piezoelectric generator.[31,32]

However, it must be borne in mind that focal hyperthermia becomes more pronounced when high-frequency shock waves are applied with the extracorporeal shock wave lithotripter Edap LT-01.[32,33]

Generally, there is a correlation between the number of shock waves and cell damage. It has also been generally observed that sensitivity to shock waves differs between different tumor cell lines, which may be a reflection of differences in their cytoskeletons, possibly causing their susceptibility to the mechanical forces associated with shock waves also to differ.

Important findings are that these effects in vitro depend on the way that cells are exposed to shock waves and can be greatly influenced by changing the conditions of the microenvironment.[28,31,32,34] Brummer reported that the L1210 mouse cell line showed severe damage when the cells were treated in suspension. However, cells immobilized in gelatin were unaffected, indicating that secondary effects are responsible for the cellular damage.[35] Smits et al[31] confirmed this observation, finding that the susceptibility of the cell lines differed between cell pellets and cell suspensions. In a cell suspension, the cytotoxicity of shock waves was more pronounced at higher cell concentrations, whereas in a pellet cytotoxicity was increased by decreasing the cell concentration.[31] The cell concentration-dependent decrease in viability may indicate that cell damage in the suspension model can be attributed to secondary shock wave effects, such as microjets, shearing force or collision, whereas in the pellet model, acceleration forces and collisions are avoided, but shock waves can have a direct impact on immobilized cells. Cavitation-related direct cytotoxicity was enhanced by reducing the cell concentration in the pellet.[31] Conversely, it has been reported that cytotoxicity in a cell suspension is independent of cell concentration.[36] In the latter experiment, cell concentration was varied fourfold whereas in the former it was varied tenfold; this may explain the discrepancy between the two sets of results.

In several experiments, shock wave-induced cytotoxicity could not be demonstrated, or was decreased after fixation of cells in gelatin.[28,31,32,34] Although the precise mechanism is not clear, it seems that this cannot be explained by the minor decrease in shock wave pressure attributable to the gelatin. However, it may be related to the cavitation phenomenon because far fewer cavitations were macroscopically observed in the gelatin medium than in medium containing no gelatin.[31] In gelatin solution, the physicoelastic properties may be altered and less cavitation may be generated. In addition, fixed cells may be less exposed to the secondary effect of shock waves such as cavitation-induced microjet streams, shearing forces and cell collision, than are cells in a pellet.

The results described above show that single-cell suspensions are not a good experimental model with which to study the cellular effects of shock waves.[32]

Combination with antitumour drugs and/or cytokines

Using single-cell suspension models, it has been shown that shock wave treatment has a potentiating effect on cytotoxic agents such as cisplatin, vinblastin, doxorubicin or 4-hydroperoxycyclophosphamide.[11,27,37–41] Similar effects on enhanced sensitivity to cytokines were also shown in the cell lines that were sensitive to the cytokines.[39] The enhanced sensitivity to drugs depended on the tumour cell line examined.

Sensitivity to cisplatin was enhanced by shock pretreatment but this effect diminished rapidly during the first hours after shock wave exposure.[39] The combined growth-inhibitory effect became most pronounced during simultaneous treatment.[39] As cisplatin cytotoxicity was not enhanced when tumour cells were exposed to shock waves after cisplatin, it was postulated that cell membrane permeability (altered cisplatin uptake and/or efflux) was altered by the shock waves.[39,40,41] Shock wave exposure could cause a transient increase in permeability of the cell membrane, thus reducing the diffusion barrier for cisplatin and increasing cisplatin influx. This interpretation was further supported by the fact that cell proliferation was enhanced following administration of a second shock wave after combined cisplatin/ shock wave treatment. A second shock-induced increase in permeability of the cell membrane after removal of the extracellular drug could increase the efflux of active cisplatin before the drug is bound to intracellular target sites, and consequently could increase the cell survival rate.[39,42]

In addition to the altered cell membrane permeability, an altered cell cycle was postulated regarding the enhanced cytotoxicity of 5-fluorouracil.[38] Further studies are necessary to disclose the mechanisms by which shock waves interact with cells and cytotoxic drugs.

Experiments in vivo

Data regarding shock wave-induced antitumour effects in vivo are controversial. Exposure to shock waves of a tumour implanted in an animal did not cause distinct histopathological or ultrastructural effects, as opposed to the findings in vitro;[27,43] however, haemorrhage and necrosis were common histopathological findings when a tumour was exposed to shock waves in vivo.[44–47]

Dose dependency

The effect of shock waves is dependent on the number of shock waves administered. In many studies, single shock waves had no effect on tumour growth; subsequently, the effect depended on the number of additional shock waves administered.[27] The growth of an N-[4-(5-nitro-2-furyl)-2-thiazolyl]formamide (FANFT)-induced bladder tumour transplanted into the leg of a mouse was not inhibited by 800 but was inhibited by 1400 shock waves.[27] Similar dose-related effects were shown with virus-induced papillomas implanted in the urinary bladder of the rabbit.[45] Dose dependency is also apparent in the finding that the smaller the initial tumour volume, the more pronounced the inhibitory effect with an equal dose of shock waves.[48] When melanoma and fibrosarcoma tumours implanted in hamsters were treated with 500–1000 shock waves/day on four consecutive days, no effect on tumour growth was noted. With the same shock wave protocol, lowering the water level over the tumour induced temporary regressions in fibrosarcomas.[49] The wave reflected from the water surface may have an important role, and this phenomenon is interpreted as an energy dose-related effect.

Tumour specificity

It has been suggested that a rapidly proliferating tumour, such as a rat prostatic tumour (which grows as a gelatinous mass, never establishing its own vascular or stromal support), generally is not suppressed by shock waves alone.[48,50–52] Studies using a rapidly growing tumour line and single-session shock wave treatment showed no effect. A rapidly metastasizing rat prostate tumour variant implanted in rats was treated by a single session of 1500 shock waves using a piezoelectric lithotripter (Piezolith 2300),[51] with no resultant reduction of tumour growth rate nor enhancement of metastatic spread. Rats with rat prostate carcinoma cells implanted in the thighs were exposed to a single session of 1000 shock waves using an electrohydraulic lithotripter,[50] with no significant change in the subsequent tumour doubling time. When subcutaneous murine bladder cancers in mice were exposed to 250–1500 shock waves alone or in combination with cisplatin,[40] shock waves alone had no effect on tumour growth; however, shock wave/cisplatin combination therapy suppressed tumour growth more than did cisplatin alone.

Less rapidly growing tumours such as human and rat kidney tumours have shown a temporary delay in growth after shock wave administration.[48] The delay in tumour growth is more prolonged when shock waves are administered repeatedly.[44] This delay is, nevertheless, temporary and several days after discontinuing shock wave administration the tumour regains its original growth potential.[44]

The tumour line dependency of the inhibitory effect of shock waves may be explained by factors related to (a) tumour doubling time,[48] (b) differences in cytoskeleton,[27] and (c) vascularization of the tumour. Well-vascularized tumours such as the NU-1 tumour are more sensitive to shock waves than are those less well vascularized, such as NC-65.[48] Shock wave-induced vascular damage and reduced tumour perfusion have been demonstrated by magnetic resonance imaging using gadolinium/diethyl-enetriamine penta-acetic acid (Gd$^+$-DTPA),[53] as well as morphologically.[47,54] Morphological changes in the kidney exposed to shock waves were characterized by renal and perirenal haemorrhage and oedema. There was endothelial cell damage in arteries, veins and glomerular capillaries,[47] and this damage was dose dependent.[54] There was indirect evidence that vascular rupture was induced by the microjets, as seen in a dog kidney in vivo.[55,56]

Combination with antitumour drugs

In most studies, shock waves combined with several chemotherapeutic drugs were apparently more effective than shock waves alone in establishing antitumour effects, although there were some small variations in the effects of the drugs.[27,40,44–46,48,52]

The enhanced therapeutic efficacy of these combined treatment modalities in vivo can be explained in several ways. First, the shock wave-induced reduction of viable tumour cells may enhance the effectiveness of chemotherapy by reducing the tumour load. Second, the impaired metabolic state of the tumour cells may render them more susceptible to chemotherapy.[57] Third, cell membrane permeability to drugs may be altered.[52] Altered metabolism of the tumour cells and increased cell membrane permeability may be induced by non-specific mechanical damage of shock waves. Fourth, the most plausible explanation is an altered blood supply caused by damage to the vasculature. The changes in local circulation may cause local accumulation of chemotherapeutic drugs. Studies on the rabbit liver in vivo have demonstrated a marked increase in local methotrexate concentrations as a result of exposure to shock waves.[32]

Summary of studies in vivo

Studies in vivo suggest that shock wave-induced tumoricidal effects mainly reflect vascular and tissue damage. Other less well-established factors include thermal and free-radical effects. Studies in vitro have shown the generation of high temperatures and the participation of cavitation-induced free radicals in cytotoxic effects, but these factors remain hypothetical in vivo. Vascular and tissue damage is induced by mechanical forces, arising from microjets (erosion), liquid flow (shearing force) and the compression and tensile forces generated at the interface of different acoustic impedances (collisions). These mechanical forces may change cell membrane permeability, alter cell metabolism[57] and make tumour cells more susceptible to antitumour drugs.

Although some authors have reported no enhancement of tumour metastasis after shock wave administration,[45,52] from the ethical standpoint these studies do not suffice for clinical application of these effects at present.

References

1. Hodgson W J B. The ultrasonic scalpel. Bull NY Acad Med 1979; 55: 908–915
2. Addonizio JC, Choudhury MS, Sayegh N. Cavitron ultrasonic surgical aspirator. Urology 1984; 25: 417–420
3. Addonizio J C, Choudhury M S. Cavitrons in urologic surgery. Urol Clin North Am 1986; 13: 435–444

4. Papachristou D N, Barters R. Resection of the liver with a water jet. Br J Surg 1982; 69: 93–94
5. Persson B G, Jeppsson B, Tranberg K-G et al. Transection of the liver with a water jet. Surg Gynecol Obstet 1989; 168: 267–268
6. Izumi R, Yabusita K, Shimizu K et al. Hepatic resection using a water jet dissector. Surg Today 1993; 23: 31–35 (in Japanese)
7. Horie T. Liver resection by water jet. Jpn J Surg 1989; 90: 82–92 (in Japanese)
8. Lingeman J E, McAteer J A, Kempson S A et al. Bioeffects of extracorporeal shock-wave lithotripsy. Urol Clin North Am 1988; 15: 507–514
9. Yokoyama M. Side effects and complication of extracorporeal shock wave lithotripsy for urolithiasis: clinical aspects. Jpn J Endourol ESWL 1993; 6: 13–28
10. Kuwahara M. Tissue injuries during extracorporeal shock wave lithotripsy from the standpoint of basic physics and experimental pathophysiology. Jpn J Endourol ESWL 1993; 6: 5–21
11. Berens M E, Welander C E, Griffin A S et al. Effect of acoustic shock waves on clonogenic growth and drug sensitivity of human tumour cells in vitro. J Urol 1989; 142: 1090–1094
12. Neppiras EA. Acoustic cavitation. Physics Rep 1980; 61: 159
13. Crum LA. The tensile strength of water. Nature 1979; 278: 148
14. Coleman A J, Saunders J E. A survey of the acoustic output of commercial extracorporeal shock wave lithotripters. Ultrasound Med Biol 1989; 15: 213–227
15. Crum L A. Cavitation microjets as a contributory mechanism for renal calculi disintegration in shock wave. J Urol 1988; 140: 1587–1590
16. Williams A R, Delius M, Miller D L et al. Investigation of cavitation in flowing media by lithotripter shock waves both in vitro and in vivo. Ultrasound Med Biol 1989; 15: 53–60
17. Coleman A, Saunders J E, Crum L et al. Acoustic cavitation generated by an extracorporeal shock wave lithotripter. Ultrasound Med Biol 1987; 13: 69–76
18. Bebjamin TB, Ellis AT. The collapse of cavitation bubbles and the pressure thereby produced against solid boundaries. Phil Trans Roy Soc Lond Ser A 1966; 260: 221–240
19. Flint E B, Suslick K S. Sonoluminescence from alkalimetal solutions. J Phys Chem 1991; 95: 1484–1488
20. Filipczynski L, Wojcik K S. The estimation of transient temperature elevation in lithotripsy and in ultrasonography. Ultrasound Med Biol 1991; 17: 715–721
21. ter Haar G R. Ultrasonic biophysics. In: Hill C R (ed) Physical principles of medical ultrasonics. Chichester: Ellis Horwood, 1986: 379–435
22. Suhr D, Bruemmer F, Huelser D F. Cavitation-generated free radicals during shock wave exposure: investigations with cell-free solutions and suspended cells. Ultrasound Med Biol 1991; 17: 761–768
23. Morgan T R, Laudone V P, Heston W D W et al. Free radical production by high energy shock waves—comparison with ionizing irradiation. J Urol 1988; 139: 186–189
24. Chaussy C, Schmiedt E, Jocham D et al. Extracorporeal shock wave lithotripsy. Basel: Karger, 1982: 8–36
25. Kambe K, Kuwahara M, Orikasa S et al. Mechanism of fragmentation of urinary stones by underwater shock wave. Urol Int 1988; 43: 275–281
26. Russo P, Stephenson R A, Mies C et al. High energy shock waves suppress tumor growth in vitro and in vivo. J Urol 1986; 135: 626–628
27. Randazzo R F, Chaussy C G, Fuchs G J et al. The in vitro and in vivo effects of extracorporeal shock waves on malignant cells. Urol Res 1988; 16: 419–426
28. Brauner T, Brummer F, Hulser D F. Histopathology of shock wave treated tumor cell suspension and multicell tumor spheroids. Ultrasound Med Biol 1989; 15: 451–460
29. Kohri K, Uemura T, Iguchi M et al. Effect of high energy shock waves on tumor cells. Urol Res 1990; 18: 101–105
30. Gambihler S, Delius M, Brendel W. Biological effects of shock waves: cell disruption, viability, and proliferation of L1210 cells exposed to shock waves in vitro. Ultrasound Med Biol 1990; 16: 587–594
31. Smits G A H, Oosterhof G O N, Ruyter A E et al. Cytotoxic effects of high energy shock wave in different in vitro models: influence of the experimental set-up. J Urol 1991; 145: 171–175

32. Jones B J, McHale A P, Butler M R. Effect of high-energy shock wave frequency on viability of malignant cell lines in vitro. Urol Res 1992; 22: 70–73

33. Vallencian G, Chopin D, Thibault P H et al. Extracorporeal focalized piezoelectric hyperthermia. Eur Urol 1990; 18(suppl 1): 285

34. McCormack D, Jones B, McElwain et al. The tumoricidal potential of extracorporeal shock wave therapy. Eur J Surg Oncol 1993; 19: 232–234

35. Brummer F, Brenner J, Brauner T et al. Effect of shock wave on suspended and immobilized L1210 cells. Ultrasound Med Biol 1989; 15: 229–239

36. van Dongen J W, van Steenbrugge G J, Romijn J C et al. The cytocidal effects of high-energy shock waves on human prostatic tumor cell lines. Eur J Clin Oncol 1989; 25: 1173–1179

37. Oosterhof G O N, Smits G A H, de Ruyter J E et al. The in vitro effect of electromagnetically generated shock waves (Lithostar) on the Dunning R3327 PAT-2 rat prostatic cancer cell-line. Urol Res 1989; 17: 13–19

38. Prat F, Sibille A, Luccioni C et al. Increased chemocytotoxicity to colon cancer cells by shock wave-induced cavitation. Gastroenterology 1994; 106: 937–944

39. Woerle K, Steinbach P, Hofstadter F. The combined effects of high-energy shock waves and cytostatic drugs or cytokines on human bladder cancer cells. Br J Cancer 1994; 69: 58–65

40. Lee K-E, Smith P, Cockett A T K. Influence of high-energy shock waves and cisplatin on antitumor effect in murine bladder cancer. Urology 1990; 26: 440–444

41. Gambihler S, Delius M. In vitro interaction of lithotripter shock waves and cytotoxic drugs. Br J Cancer 1992; 66: 69–73

42. Melvik J E, Dornish J M, Pettersen E O. The binding of cis-dichlorodiamineplatinum(II) to extracellular and intracellular components in relation to drug uptake and cytotoxicity in vitro. Br J Cancer 1992; 66: 260–265

43. Russo P, Mies C, Huryk R et al. Histopathologic and ultrastructural correlations of tumor growth suppression by high energy shock waves. J Urol 1987; 137: 338–341

44. Oosterhof G O N, Smits G A H, de Ruyter J E et al. Effect of high-energy shock waves combined with biological response modifiers or Adriamycin on a human kidney cancer xenograft. Urol Res 1990; 18: 419–424

45. Hoshi S, Orikasa S, Kuwahara M et al. High energy underwater shock wave treatment on implanted urinary bladder cancer in rabbits. J Urol 1991; 146: 439–443

46. Hoshi S, Orikasa S, Kuwahara M et al. Shock wave and THP–Adriamycin for treatment of rabbit's bladder cancer. Jpn J Cancer Res 1992; 83: 248–250

47. Karlsen S J, Smevick B, Hovig T. Acute morphological changes in canine kidneys after exposure to extracorporeal shock waves. Urol Res 1991; 19: 105–115

48. Oosterhof G O N, Smits G A H, de Ruyter A E et al. In vivo effect of high energy shock waves on urological tumors: an evaluation of treatment modalities. J Urol 1990; 144: 785–789

49. Weiss N, Delius M, Gambihler S et al. Influence of the shock wave application mode on the growth of A-MEL 3 and SSK2 tumors in vivo. Ultrasound Med Biol 1990; 16: 595–605

50. Laudone V P, Morgan T R, Huryk R F et al. Cytotoxicity of high energy shock waves: methodological consideration. J Urol 1989; 141: 965–968

51. Geldof A A, De Voogt H J, Rao B R. High energy shock waves do not affect either primary tumor growth or metastasis of prostate carcinoma, R3327-MatLyLu. Urol Res 1989; 17: 9–12

52. Holmes R P, Yeaman L I, Li W-J et al. The combined effects of shock waves and cisplatin therapy on rat prostate tumors. J Urol 1990; 144: 159–163

53. Gamarra F, Naegele M, Lumper W et al. Acute effect of shock waves on tumors assessed by magnetic resonance imaging. Possible role of blood flow reduction. Invest Radiol 1993; 28: 611–618

54. Delius M, Enders G, Xuan Z et al. Biological effects of shock waves: kidney damage by shock waves in dog—dose dependence. Ultrasound Med Biol 1988; 14: 117–122

55. Ioritani N, Kuwahara M, Kambe K et al. Renal tissue damage induced by focused shock waves. Am Inst Physics Conf Proc 1990; 208: 185–190

56. Kuwahara M, Ioritani N, Kambe K et al. Hyperechoic region induced by focused shock waves in vitro and in vivo: possibility of acoustic cavitation bubbles. J Lithotripsy Stone Dis 1990; 1: 282–288

57. Smits G A H, Heerschap A, Oosterhof G O N et al. Early metabolic response to high energy shock waves in a human tumor kidney xenograft monitored by 31P magnetic resonance spectroscopy. Ultrasound Med Biol 1991; 17: 791–801
58. Yahiro T. Review of the jet cutting technology in Japan. Int Conf Geomechanics 91, Czechoslovakia, September 1991.

Microscopic and macroscopic study of the effects of thermotherapy

2

B. Mauroy   M. Chive   D. Demetriou   B. Hattab
J. P. Sozanski   F. Callot   F. Carpentier   J. Biserte
E. Mazeman

Introduction

One of the main problems in thermotherapy of the prostate is still that of thermometry, because implanted thermoprobes (thermocouples or optical fibres), which provide only temperature data limited to a small volume of tissue around the measuring point, cannot be used easily during the heating session: only rectal or urethral surface catheter thermoprobes are generally used. The problem has finally been solved by using microwave radiometry, which enables total temperature control of the heated tissue to be obtained, and in which the same applicator antenna operates the heating and the radiometric temperature measurement.[1-4]

The Prostcare apparatus (Bruker Spectospin, Wissembourg, France), which is a microwave thermotherapy system for treatment of benign prostatic hyperplasica, (BPH), with a radiometer for intraprostatic temperature control, was used for clinical experiments.

Materials and methods

Prostcare system

This allows treatment of the prostate by the urethral or the endorectal route; in the study described here, only the former route was used. This thermotherapy apparatus comprises a 915 MHz microwave generator delivering variable power, a 3 GHz microwave radiometer for temperature measurement, a urethral applicator (for heating and radiometry) made of a coaxial antenna introduced within the Foley-type plastic catheter and maintained at a constant temperature of 20°C by water flowing into the catheter, plus a computer to regulate the thermotherapy session.

The system operates according to the alternate method, i.e. heating is achieved at any time whereas radiometric temperature measurement takes place for 8 s each minute when the generator is switched off.

Applicator antenna and temperature measurement by radiometry

The microwave antenna is made from a flexible coaxial cable, 2 mm in external diameter, of 50 Ω characteristic impedance. At the end of this coaxial cable the external conductor has been removed over a length h to produce a radiating antenna of active length equal to $2h$. This length has been optimized in order to transfer at least 90% of the 915 MHz microwave energy to the prostate volume to be heated. This antenna is also used for radiometry as an antenna receiver for temperature measurement.[1-3]

The physical basis of radiometry is the fact that a given body, the temperature of which is raised to 0 K, emits spontaneous electromagnetic radiation of thermal origin—so-called thermal noise power. Because this noise power is directly related to the body temperature, measurement of the emitted thermal power using a radiometer gives information about that temperature. When the noise power collected by the antenna and the radiometer centred on 3 GHz (with 1 GHz bandwidth) is measured, this thermal noise power which results from heating of the prostate is the integral summation of the elementary noise power emitted by each subvolume in the prostate volume coupled to the antenna in the frequency range of the radiometer. Thus, the radiometer gives temperature data corresponding to the average temperature of the entire volume of prostate tissue heated.

Principle of the clinical study

Thermotherapy was applied to ten patients who each had a large prostate adenoma requiring prostatectomy. After general anaesthesia, the thermo-therapy catheter was inserted and the balloon was inflated to 30 ml and positioned in the bladder neck. The microwave antenna was then introduced into the catheter and firmly fixed to it in the defined position, preventing any displacement during the heating session. Antenna and catheter were then connected to the microwave generator and to the thermostatically controlled water bag, respectively.

A four-point optical fibre was implanted in the prostate to obtain comparative data for radiometric and optical fibre point temperature measurements during the heating session.

For three patients in this series, two optical fibres were implanted in the adenoma after the bladder had been opened. Each thermoprobe was implanted within 5 mm of the bladder neck, in order to be as parallel as possible to the urethra, which proved difficult given the slant of this section of the urethra. Radiographic assessment showed that opening the bladder was not necessary and that the catheter could be implanted through the prostate capsule. The other seven patients in this series had only one thermoprobe implanted.

In both groups, intraprostatic temperature was measured during the heating session by radiometry, and continuously throughout the entire session by thermoprobes. The heating sessions initially lasted for 1 h but, in view of the results achieved, the last four patients in the series received heating for 30 min (15 min heating proved insufficient).

Ten minutes after the end of the heating session, adenomectomy was performed, in the first three cases through the transvesical route and in the other cases through the retropubic route. The adenomas weighed between 50 and 180 g. The study of each adenoma comprised macroscopic assessment (and photographs) of the adenoma, histological analysis (always on the same transverse plane) and correlation between the macroscopic and microscopic lesions found and the heating curves.

No specific complications (haemorrhagic in particular) were observed either before or after operation.

Results

Measurement of temperature delivered to the prostate

Temperatures were measured and recorded during the thermotherapy sessions using the radiometer and the four-point (F1–F4) optical fibre (Fig. 2.1). F1 and F2, located 4–5 mm from the catheter in the prostate zone where the microwave power deposition is maximum, indicated very high temperatures (55–60°C). F3 (about 15 mm from the catheter) and F4 (about 25 mm from the catheter) located outside this hot zone showed temperatures of 46 and 41°C, respectively.

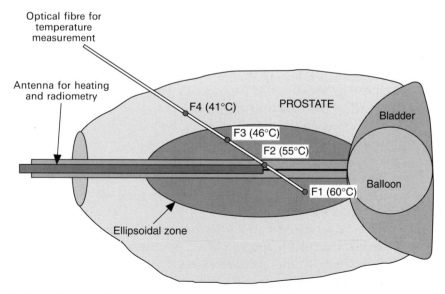

Fig. 2.1. Diagram of location of four-point optical fibre in the prostate during thermotherapy [distance from the urethra, 4–5 mm (F1, F2), 15 mm (F3) and 25 mm (F4)]. The ellipsoidal zone corresponds to the volume of prostate tissue heated by microwave power emitted by the antenna (915 MHz); it is this volume that contributes to the radiometric signal ('radiometric temperature').

The radiometer gives the average temperature of all the volume heated, including the hot spots (F1, F2) and the low zones (F3, F4), and therefore indicates the so-called radiometer temperature, 45–47°C. This radiometer temperature is the mean temperature delivered to the prostate, compared with the point measurements given by the optical fibre.

Histological lesions

The macroscopic and microscopic aspect varied with the temperature delivered at the prostate. For a radiometric temperature of 47°C, as administered to eight patients, macroscopic assessment showed the presence of ellipsoidal periurethral necrosis. In these cases, microscopic examination revealed spread of the necrosis (a) to the urethral epithelium, which was desquamated and replaced with fibrinous masses, (b) to the subjacent connective tissue, which showed recent fibrinous thromboses, (c) to the smooth muscle fibres, which were damaged, with dense pyknotic nuclei, and (d) to the prostatic glands, the last to be affected with desquamation of the gland epithelium. Necrosis usually spreads in the first three of these components and sometimes goes deeply into the smooth muscle fibres, spreading between glandular lobuli that are as yet undamaged. This type of necrosis was, indeed, identified in all eight patients; it was situated in the periurethral region and was ellipsoidal in shape, forming a periurethral sheath 30 mm long and 10–20 mm wide on either side of the urethra. As an example, Fig. 2. shows the necrotic areas in one patient; the shape and volume of necrosis was identical in the eight patients heated to a radiometric thermal level of 47°C.

Discussion

This clinical study was designed to ascertain which lesions are induced by thermotherapy, whether necrosis can be induced and if so by what thermal levels, and whether this technique can be reproduced—in other words, what is the most reliable way of inducing necrosis.

Lesions induced by thermotherapy

The lesions induced vary with the temperature delivered to the prostate.

In the series of ten patients, the first patient only received heating for 1 h at a thermal radiometric level of 44°C. At this temperature, when the adenoma was opened the mucosa showed only haemorrhagic dots. Histological examination revealed two types of lesions: (1) obvious vasodilation of the mucosa, with haemorrhagic suffusion; and (2) medium-sized inflammatory infiltrates that were difficult to interpret, given the presence of an adenoma. Only a few muscle fibres were affected; their nuclei were small, dense and pyknotic.

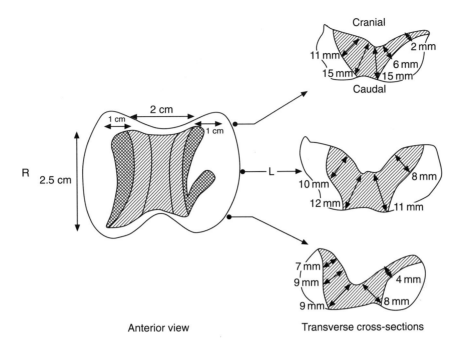

Fig. 2.2. Necrotic area of prostate after heating (patient no. 3).

Another adenoma in this series, which had received a thermal radiometric level of 46°C, displayed the same macroscopic aspect, but histological examination revealed necrotic lesions that were shallower than those in the other patients, who had received a thermal radiometric level of 47°C.

Finally, a thermal radiometric level of 47°C (which corresponds to a temperature of 55–60°C when measured by implanted optical fibres) delivered to the prostate invariably induces identical necrotic lesions, as observed in eight patients in this study.

Which thermal levels induce necrosis?

After it was noted that a thermal radiometric level of 47°C induced necrosis, the apparatus was set at this temperature. In eight patients, this radiometric temperature (which corresponds to an intraprostatic temperature of 55–60°C) induced ellipsoidal periurethral necrosis, comprising desquamation of the urethral epithelium, intravascular fibrinous thromboses in the subjacent connective tissue and a few areas of haemorrhagic suffusion, degeneration of the smooth muscle fibres with nuclear pyknosis, and degeneration and desquamation of the cells of the glandular epithelium. These alterations in the cells and tissues affect the normal prostatic structures as well as those that are hyperplastic and adenomatous, but adenomatous prostatic structures undergo less internal degeneration than do non-adenomatous prostatic tissues.

The histological lesions observed always correspond to a coagulative necrosis. The importance of these lesions was assessed initially by macroscopic examination of serial prostatic cross-sections, and subsequently by microscopic examination of samples of these sections. This enabled the extent of necrosis (width and length) to be established precisely (Table 2.1). The necrotic shaft was ellipsoidal with an average length of 25–30 mm, approximately the length of the adenoma; on either side of the urethral lumen the necrotic lesions were 15–20 mm wide (Fig. 2.2).

There were six 1 h heating sessions; the heating time was then reduced to 45 min in one case and to 30 min in two cases. The lesions had exactly the same macroscopic and microscopic aspect after a 30 min heating session.

Can this necrosis be reproduced?

The efficacy of thermotherapy is related to the rapidity of the increase in microwave power. The results of this clinical study have enabled the following protocol to be drawn up:

1. At the beginning of the heating session the desired radiometric level is set at 47°C.
2. During the first minute of heating, 55 W are delivered by the antenna to the prostate.
3. In the second minute 60 W are applied, then 65 W during the third minute and 70 W for the fourth minute.
4. After each minute of heating, the generator is switched off and the temperature is measured radiometrically for 8 s.

This protocol induces a very rapid temperature increase, attaining a thermal radiometric level of 47–48°C in 3 min. This limits the vascularization phenomena in the prostate and creates a region of high temperature (>50°C) 5–6 mm wide in the prostate around the urethra, causing necrosis of the prostatic tissues. After 4 min heating the power is automatically reduced by the computer on the basis of the radiometric temperature measurements in order to maintain a temperature of 47–48°C in the prostate during the desired heating time (60 min or less).

Figure 2.3 depicts an example of this technical protocol and shows the power emitted and radiometric temperature over time for two patients.

Conclusions

This chapter is concerned with the immediate consequences of

Patient no.	Radiometric temperature (°C)	Intraprostatic temperature (°C)	Duration of heating (min)	Lesion		
				Histological lesions	Height (mm)	Width around urethra, top–middle–bottom
1	44	46–48	60	Haemorrhagic suffusion + inflammatory infiltrates	30	2–5–4
2	46	48–50	60	Coagulative necrosis	45	4–6–5
3	47	55–60	60	Coagulative necrosis	45	25–30–20
4	47	55–60	60	Coagulative necrosis	40	19–25–28
5	47	55–60	60	Coagulative necrosis	45	30–43–25
6	47	55–60	60	Coagulative necrosis	43	23–30–25
7	47	55–60	45	Coagulative necrosis	30	25–45–27
8	47	55–60	45	Coagulative necrosis	35	20–25–12
9	47	55–60	30	Coagulative necrosis	35	25–30–20
10	47	55–60	30	Coagulative necrosis	60	14–18–13

Table 2.1. Extent of periurethral necrosis in ten patients receiving thermotherapy

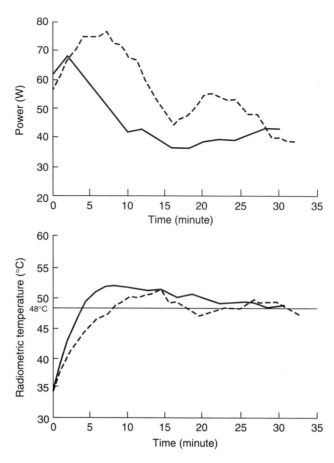

Fig. 2.3. Microwave power emitted and radiometric temperature over a 30 min period of thermotherapy for patients 4 (——) and 9 (– – –).

thermotherapy. Research is currently under way to assess its subsequent effects, which are undoubtedly more important. Six weeks after the treatment described above, endoscopic examination of these patients, who did not undergo surgery, showed the existence of adenomatous necrosis and intratumoral cavities. Further investigations of the consequences of thermotherapy followed by adenomectomy 72 h, 3 weeks, 6 weeks or 3 months later, is currently under way.

The following are necessary for effective thermotherapy (with temperature measurement by radiometry):

1. Radiometric temperature of 47°C (55–60°C delivered to the prostate).
2. Minimum 30 min duration of each session to ensure efficacy.
3. A rapid increase in power, reaching 80 W in 5 min maximum. As soon as necrosis is obtained, the power is automatically reduced.

References

1. Chive M. Use of microwave radiometry for hyperthermia monitoring and as a basis for thermal dosimetry. In: Methods of hyperthermia control. Clinical Thermology series (subseries Thermotherapy). Berlin: Springer Verlag, 1990: 3; 113–128
2. Chive M, Belot G, Mabire JP et al. Applications of a microwave hyperthermia system controlled by microwave radiometry for the treatment of BPH. Proc 6th Int Congr Hyperthermia Oncol 1992; 1: 461
3. Fabre JJ, Chive M, Dubois JC. 915 MHz microwave interstitial hyperthermia. Part I: Theoretical and experimental aspects with temperature control by multifrequency radiometry. Int J Hyperthermia 1993; 9: 433–444
4. Belot G, Chive M. Transurethral thermotherapy of benign prostate hypertrophy controlled by radiometry. Eur Urol 1993; 23: 326–329

Is hyperthermia a valuable therapy for BPH? Results of a double-blind randomized study

3

C.-C. Abbou   C. Payan   C. Viens-Bitker   F. Richard
L. Boccon-Gibod   A. Jardin   D. Beurton   A. Le Duc
J. Fermanian—French BPH Hyperthermia Group

Introduction

Benign prostatic hyperplasia (BPH) is a common disease in ageing men.[1] Its frequency and cost of treatment make this disease a real public health problem.[2,3]

Symptoms are independent of prostatic volume[4] and may fluctuate and even resolve spontaneously.[5,6] It follows that the placebo effect of any treatment may be significant and that objective endpoints must be used to determine treatment efficacy.

Currently accepted objective criteria for assessing BPH and evaluating response to therapy include urinary flow rate and voided volume, prostatic volume and residual urine.[7,8] In addition, subjective parameters (symptom scores) are used to assess the quality of life.[9] However, the evaluation of therapy remains difficult, as an improvement in symptoms alone does not imply that therapeutic objectives have been met; furthermore, the absence of improvement in objective symptoms may be well tolerated.[4]

Because surgical procedures can induce complications,[10] particularly in older and debilitated patients, several strategies for the conservative management of BPH have been developed.

Recently, hyperthermia created by microwaves has been used to treat BPH. Although heat has been demonstrated to cause cell death in tumour tissue,[11] this effect has not been reported in BPH. Reported results are conflicting: some show improvement in objective and subjective criteria in patients who could have been candidates for surgery,[12–17] but other authors are less optimistic about this type of treatment, finding no improvement in objective criteria or, at best, the equivalent of a placebo effect.[18–21] After preliminary results given by Devonec et al,[22] thermotherapy using temperatures over 45°C appears to give significant improvements in terms of peak flow rate (PFR) and the Madsen score at 3 months. To assess the ef-fectiveness of hyperthermia on BPH, a double-blind randomized multicentre clinical trial was conducted. The aim was to compare the safety and efficacy of hyperthermia with a sham group, taking into account the approach (transrectal or transurethral).

Patients and methods

Seven urological departments contributed to the recruitment of patients with symptomatic prostatism.

Selection criteria

Inclusion criteria were as follows: age over 50; voiding disorders for at least 3 months (prior to the study); no suspicion of prostatic cancer (rectal examination); prostatic weight ranging from 30 to 80 g, as assessed by transrectal ultrasound using the elliptical method or the simplified formula based on the diameters of three dimensions [weight=(sagittal × axial × coronal)/2]; PFR less than 15 ml/s for a voided volume of 150 ml or more, determined by two urine flow measurements; residual urine volume less than 300 ml (suprapubic ultrasound on two different days); intravenous pyelogram (IVP) with a cystourethrogram; prostate-specific antigen (PSA) less than 10 ng/ml (assessed by radioimmunoassay, RIA) for a prostate weighing less than 60 g or PSA less than 15 ng/ml for a prostate weighing 60 g or more; serum creatinine of less than 160 μmol/l; lack of infection (bacter-iological analysis of urine); and written informed consent from each patient.

Non-inclusion criteria were previous surgery on the prostate or bladder; mental incapacity; any chronic disease potentially hindering follow-up; diabetes; participation in any clinical protocol within the last 3 months; any other urological disease; any medical treatment for voiding disorders within 15 days of inclusion; diuretics in the previous 3 months; anticoagulant therapy; allergy to lidocaine; and colorectal disease.

Randomization

Randomization was done by a single treatment centre after verification of the inclusion criteria; it was stratified by the investigating centre and according to approach (transrectal or transurethral). Randomization was done using permutation tables, and was designed to obtain each type of approach, for equal sample sizes for each device and sham group. The number of patients per group (n=70) was calculated according to the following hypothesis: 50% response rate in each hyperthermia group and 20% in each sham group, with x and y risks of 5%.

Treatment

Three different devices were used for transrectal treatment (Biodan, Brucker, Tecnomatix) and three for transurethral treatment (Direx, Bruker, BSD). Temperature was monitored by an integrated microwave generator and controlled in each device through a fibre-optic temperature monitor. The frequency (one session for the transurethral treatment and six sessions over 3 weeks for the transrectal treatment) and duration (1–3 h for each session) of treatment sessions depended on the device used. Sham treatment consisted of a single session with temperature kept at 37°C. All patients were treated in a single treatment centre.

Evaluations

Patients were evaluated at 3, 6 and 12 months. During the treatment period and early follow-up (1 and 4 weeks after treatment) any complications were noted.

For each patient the response was assessed separately according to subjective (Madsen score) and objective (PFR) criteria. The principal analysis was done after 12 months of follow-up. Excellent, good and moderate responses were defined according to the final value (Madsen score, PFR) and percentage of change from baseline (Table 3.1). As treatment response rates were low, the excellent, good and moderate responses were combined to analyse the effect of treatment. Thus, for this analysis, 'Responders' are patients showing excellent, good or moderate responses according to each criterion analysed separately (Madsen score

(a) Subjective

Treatment response	Subjective
No response	Madsen score > 5 and/or decrease ratio < 30%
Moderate	Madsen score ⩾ 5 with a decrease ratio of 30–50%
Good	Madsen score < 5 with a decrease ratio of 30–50% or
	Madsen score ⩾ 5 with a decrease ratio ⩾ 50%
Excellent	Madsen score < 5 with a decrease ratio ⩾ 50%

(b) Objective

Treatment response	Objective
No response	PFR* < 10 ml/s, or between 10 and 15 with an increase < 30%
Moderate	PFR between 10 and 15 ml/s with an increase of 30–50%
Good	PFR ⩾ 15 ml/s with an increase between 30 and 50% or PFR between 10 and 15 ml/s with increase ⩾ 50%
Excellent	PFR ⩾ 15 ml/s with an increase > 50%

Table 3.1 Response criteria

*PFR, peak flow rate.

decrease of more than 30%; PFR more than 10 ml/s with PFR increase of more than 30%). 'Non-responders' are patients who dropped out during treatment (because of complications or complementary treatment, or who refused to continue) and patients who did not show a response to treatment (Madsen score decrease of less than 30%; PFR less than 10 ml/s or PFR of more than 10 ml/s with an increase of less than 30%).

Patients lost to follow-up were classified according to maximum bias (in the sham groups as 'Responder' and in the hyperthermia groups as 'Non-responder').

Statistical methods

Data were checked before analysis by an independent clinical study unit (Comité d'évaluation et de diffusion des innovations technologiques).

The chi-square test was used to compare independent proportions between groups, and Student's t test (or the Mann–Whitney test when normality could not be assumed) to compare means between groups.

Multiple logistic regression was used to determine which covariates explained the outcome (response, or no response) of treatment. To verify the comparability of the results obtained with the different devices, the response rates were first compared for each type of approach (transrectal or transurethral); as no difference was found in either case, the results for each approach were combined. An overall logistic analysis was then performed with the following covariates: treatment approach, interaction between treatment according to approach, and baseline PFR—a variable which differed significantly (Student's t test) between the responders and non-responders.

All tests were two-tailed and the threshold of significance was set at $p < 0.05$. The BMDP software program was used for the statistical analysis.

Results

A total of 226 patients were randomized: 16 opted not to be treated (12 in the transrectal hyperthermia group and four in the sham group). Ten treated patients were excluded from the analysis before decoding (nine patients with voided volume of less than 150 ml and residual urine of less than 100 ml and one with no baseline flow-rate measurement). Thus, 200 treated patients were evaluated (131 hyperthermia, 69 sham).

There were no significant differences in baseline characteristics between the sham and treated groups within each type of approach (Table 3.2).

Complications during treatment (Table 3.3)

No complications were observed during treatment in the sham groups. Fewer patients had complications during treatment in the transurethral

	Transurethral route		Transrectal route	
Parameter	Hyperthermia (n=66)	Sham (n=31)	Hyperthermia (n=65)	Sham (n=38)
Age	65±8	66±7	66±7	66±7
Madsen score	10.9±4.3	12.8±4.5	11.7±4.3	12.1±4.5
PFR* (ml/s)	10.4±2.7	9.9±2.5	9.8±2.7	9.0±3.3
Prostate weight (g)	45±15	44±11	45±13	43±15
Voided volume (ml)	249±82	242±89	231±84	219±72
Residual urine (ml)	66±60	61±42	79±55	61±55
Micturition time (s)	52±24	59±24	54±22	61±36
PSA†	4.5±2.7	4.2±3.0	4.8±2.8	5.0±3.3
Creatinine (µmol/l)	100±19	92±16	92±19	90±19

Table 3.2. Baseline characteristics (mean±SD) of 200 patients given transurethral or transrectal hyperthermia or the corresponding sham treatment

*PFR, peak flow rate; †PSA, prostate-specific antigen.

group than in the transrectal group ($p<0.0001$). Four patients (6%) in the transurethral group had complications (two cases of urethral bleeding, one of acute retention and one in which treatment was interrupted because of pain). In the transrectal hyperthermia group, 22 patients (34%) had side effects during or between treatment sessions, and 11 decided not to

	Groups		
Complication	Transurethral (n=66)	Transrectal (n=65)	Shams (n=69)
Urethral bleeding	2 (3)*	13 (20)	0
Urethral pain	1 (1.5)	5 (8)	0
Rectal pain	0	8 (12.3)	0
Acute retention	1 (1.5)	1 (1.5)	0
Faecal incontinence	0	1 (1.5)	0
Chest or hypogastric pain	0	5 (7.6)	0
Tachycardia	0	1 (1.5)	0
Fainting	0	1 (1.5)	0
Total no. of complications	4	35	0
Total no. of patients	4 (6)†	22 (34)	0
Drop-outs during treatment	1 (1.5)	11 (17)	0

Table 3.3. Complications during treatment

*Percentages in parentheses; †transurethral<transrectal, $p<0.01$.

continue treatment. The main complications were urethral bleeding and rectal pain.

Early post-treatment complications (Table 3.4)

More patients had complications during the 4 weeks following treatment in the transurethral hyperthermia group than in the transrectal group ($p < 0.001$), and than in the sham groups ($p < 0.05$). Urethral bleeding and cystitis were the main complications.

Complication	Transurethral route		Transrectal route	
	Hyperthermia (n=66)	Sham (n=31)	Hyperthermia (n=65)	Sham (n=38)
Urethral bleeding	18 (27)*	9 (29)	7 (11)	5 (13)
Cystitis	12 (18)	6 (19)	2 (3)	4 (11)
Acute retention	0	0	1 (1.5)	0
Haemospermia	0	0	6 (9)	0
Urinary tract infection	0	1 (3)	0	0
Prostatitis	1 (1.5)	1 (3)	0	0
Other	4 (6)	0	6 (9)	4 (11)
Total no. of complications	35	17	22	13
Total no. of patients	30 (45)†	11 (35)	12 (18)	9 (24)

Table 3.4. Early complications after treatment

*Percentages in parentheses; †transurethral hyperthermia>transrectal hyperthermia, $p<0.001$.

Drop-outs during follow-up

Drop-outs during follow-up represented 17% in the transurethral group, 23% in the transrectal group and 38% and 13%, respectively, in the sham groups. Drop-outs during follow-up were mainly due to complementary medical or surgical treatment for worsening obstructive symptoms; medical treatment was more frequent in the hyperthermia groups, whereas patients in the sham group underwent surgical treatment more frequently. Only two patients were lost to follow-up (one in the transurethral sham group and one in the transrectal hyperthermia group).

All drop-outs were included in the analysis at 12 months as non-responders, except for two patients who were excluded for reasons unrelated to treatment.

Overall results

The efficacy of hyperthermia was evaluated at 12 months according to the above-mentioned criteria (Table 3.1). As treatment response rates were low, the moderate, good and excellent responses were combined in one 'Response' category.

When outcome was assessed according to PFR, no significant predicting covariate was found in the logistic regression analysis. When outcome was considered in terms of the Madsen score, the only significant covariate was the treatment × approach interaction (logistic coefficient=2.45, $p=0.0004$), suggesting that the treatment effect differs in the two approaches (rectal and urethral).

For this reason, the results for each type of approach are presented separately. As shown in Table 3.5, objective response rates were low (less than 20% in all the groups). There was no significant difference in objective response rates between the transrectal approach versus the corresponding sham and the transurethral compared with its sham. Subjective responses were significantly better only in the transurethral group compared with its sham (50% vs 17%, $p<0.01$). Furthermore, no significant difference was found between the mean improvement over baseline (PFR and Madsen score).

Response	Transurethral route			Transrectal route		
	Hyperthermia (n=66)	Sham (n=29)	p value	Hyperthermia (n=65)	Sham (n=38)	p value
Objective (PFR*) (%)	14	17	NS†	8	16	NS
Subjective (Madsen score) (%)	50	17	$p<0.01$	25	39	NS

Table 3.5. Objective and subjective results at 1 year in Sham, transurethral and transrectal groups
*PFR, peak flow rate; †NS, not significant.

Results were analysed at 3 and 6 months. Again, no significant difference in PFR response rates emerged between the hyperthermia and sham groups, and the rates of response were as low as at 12 months. Madsen score response rates did not vary with time in the transurethral hyperthermia group, but fell slightly in the sham and transrectal groups.

Discussion

Initial trials of transrectal and transurethral hyperthermia showed promising results in the treatment of BPH[12,23,24] and later reports suggested that hyperthermia was a potential non-surgical alternative for the treatment of symptomatic BPH. However, clinical studies using both the transrectal and transurethral approach showed varying effects on objective and subjective symptoms. Because of the multiplicity of microwave hyperthermia devices and the paucity of randomized trials, it remains difficult to define the ultimate role of hyperthermia in BPH.

In a recent prospective randomized study, Zerbib et al[12] compared transrectal hyperthermia with sham treatment (one hyperthermia session weekly for 5 weeks at 43°C). Although patients were evaluated at 3 months only, this study showed objective and subjective improvements in the treatment group compared with the sham group. In contrast, in sham-controlled studies using transrectal hyperthermia, Fabricius et al[25] and Strohmaier et al[19] reported no objective difference between the two groups, although subjective differences did emerge. In addition, these studies suggested that the placebo effect improved symptoms in about 30% of cases.[12]

Transurethral hyperthermia appears to be able to increase the temperature to more than 42°C in symmetrical volumes of up to 5 cm^3, and to provide penetration of heat to a depth of 0.5 cm around the probe.[26] Preliminary reports using transurethral hyperthermia support the view that direct heating is more effective for the treatment of obstructive symptoms than is the transrectal approach.[27] Although the transurethral approach was effective in the treatment of symptomatic BPH, particularly in terms of subjective symptoms [US Food and Drug Administration (FDA) severity score], prostate volume, post-voiding residual volume and PFR did not differ from those in patients treated with transrectal hyperthermia.[27] Furthermore, in a large prospective Canadian study,[16] objective criteria improved in 78% and symptoms in 83% of treated patients. It is not clear whether this effect is durable, as in most of these reports the follow-up period was short. However, the effect of hyperthermia may not, in fact, be durable, as exacerbation of symptoms occurs in patients who initially respond to therapy.[27]

This study was designed to follow the guidelines issued by the Association Française d'Urologie (AFU) for the investigation of alternative treatments for BPH. The parameters used to define objective and subjective responses are similar to those recommended by the FDA. Guidelines for the clinical investigation of devices used for the treatment of BPH have since become available. This study enabled the sham effect to be estimated and the effects of transurethral and transrectal hyperthermia to be compared.

This double-blind randomized study showed no objective response at 12 months follow-up with either the transrectal or the transurethral approach. Only transurethral treatment gave better results than the corresponding sham on the subjective Madsen score, with 50% versus 17% of responders, respectively ($p < 0.01$).

Unequal sizes of treatment and sham groups (because of randomization between several devices) induces no bias but could lead to a lack of statistical power.

There are a number of possible reasons for the conflicting results reported in the literature using transrectal and transurethral hyperthermia in BPH. The most obvious is the choice of endpoints. In this study, the effectiveness of hyperthermia was defined by specific criteria including subjective and objective response goals, rather than an improvement in the mean values of these criteria. In addition, patients who dropped out of the study for reasons related to treatment were considered as non-responders.

In the light of this and previous studies, the authors consider that hyperthermia is not an effective treatment for BPH, nor is it an alternative to transurethral prostatectomy. However, the symptomatic improvement in the transurethral group of patients in this study seems to warrant a long-term trial (at least 12 months) of hyperthermia compared with medical therapy.

Acknowledgements

This study was supported by a grant from the Comité d'Evaluation et de Diffusion des Innovations Technologiques (CEDIT), Assistance Publique, Hôpitaux de Paris. Devices were lent by the following companies: Biodan, Brucker, BSD, Direx and Tecnomatix.

References

1. Isaacs J T. Importance of the natural history of benign prostatic hyperplasia in the evaluation of pharmacologic intervention. Prostate 1990; 3(suppl): 1S–7S
2. Garraway W M, Collins G N, Lee R J. High prevalence of benign prostatic hypertrophy in the community. Lancet 1991; 338: 469–471
3. Drummond M F, McGuire A J, Black N A et al. Economic burden of treated benign prostatic hyperplasia in the United Kingdom. Br J Urol 1993; 71: 290–296
4. Andersen J T. Benign prostatic hyperplasia: symptoms and objective assessment. Eur Urol 1991; 20(suppl 2): 36S–40S
5. Craigen A A, Hickling J B, Saunders C R G, Carpentier R G. Natural history of prostatic obstruction. J Roy Coll Gen Pract 1969; 18: 226–232
6. Uson A C, Paez A B, Uson-Jaeger J. The natural history and course of untreated BPH. Eur J Urol 1991; 20(suppl 2): 22S–26S
7. Badlani G H. Preoperative evaluation in benign prostatic hyperplasia. J Endourol 1991; 5: 169–174
8. Cucchi A. Urinary uroflow rate in benign prostatic hypertrophy in relation to the degree of obstruction of the vesical outlet. Br J Urol 1992; 69: 272–276
9. Barry M J, Fowler F J. O'Leary M P et al. Correlation of the American Urological Association Index with self administered versions of the Madsen–Iversen, Boyarsky and Maine Medical Assessment Program Symptom Indexes. J Urol 1992; 148: 1558–1563
10. Mebust W K, Holtgrewe H L, Cockett A T K, Peters P C. Transurethral prostatectomy: immediate and postoperative complications. A cooperative study of 13 participating institutions evaluating 3,885 patients. J Urol 1989; 141: 243–247
11. Overgaard J. Effect of hyperthermia on malignant cells in vivo: a review and a hypothesis. Cancer 1979, 43: 767–782

12. Zerbib M, Steg A, Conquy S et al. Localized hyperthermia versus the sham procedure in obstructive benign hyperplasia of the prostate: a prospective randomized study. J Urol 1992; 147: 1048–1052

13. Baert O, Ameye F, Willemen P et al. Transurethral microwave hyperthermia for benign prostatic hyperplasia: preliminary clinical and pathological results. J Urol 1990; 144: 1383–1387

14. Okada K, Yoshida T, Endo M et al. Significance of transrectal hyperthermia in the treatment of benign prostatic hyperplasia. Jpn J Urol 1991; 82: 455–461 (in Japanese)

15. Serrate Aguilera R, Ruis Espina G, Regie Aldosa R et al. Local hyperthermia in the treatment of benign prostatic hyperplasia. Assessment of 100 patients. Eur Urol 1991; 20: 9–11

16. Le May C. First Canadian clinical study of transurethral hyperthermia in benign prostatic hyperplasia. Assessment of 220 patients. Eur Urol 1992; 21: 184–186

17. Yerushalmi A, Singer D, Katsnelson R et al. Localised deep microwave hyperthermia in the treatment of benign prostatic hyperplasia: long-term assessment. Br J Urol 1992; 70: 178–192

18. Saranga R, Matzkin H, Braf Z. Local microwave hyperthermia in the treatment of benign prostatic hypertrophy. Br J Urol 1990; 65: 349–353

19. Strohmaier W L, Bichler KH, Fluchter SH, Wilbert DM. Local microwave hyperthermia of benign prostatic hyperplasia. J Urol 1990; 144: 913–917

20. Bichler K H, Strohmaier W L, Fluchter S H. Local hyperthermia in benign prostatic hyperplasia. Urologe A 1991; 30: 122–126 (in German)

21. Montorsi F, Galli L, Guazzoni G et al. Transrectal microwave hyperthermia for benign prostatic hyperplasia: long-term clinical, pathological and ultrastructural patterns. J Urol 1992; 148: 321–325

22. Devonec M, Ogden C, Perrin P, St Clair Carter S. Clinical response to transurethral microwave thermotherapy is thermal dose dependent. Eur Urol 1993; 23: 267–274

23. Servadio C. Local hyperthermia for the treatment of prostatic disease. In: Fitzpatrick J M, Krane K (eds) The prostate. New York: Churchill Livingstone, 1986; 223–228

24. Servadio C, Leib Z, Lev A. Further observation on the use of local hyperthermia for the treatment of disease of the prostate in man. Eur Urol 1986; 12: 101

25. Fabricius P G, Schafer J, Schmeller N. Efficacy of transrectal hyperthermia for benign prostatic hyperplasia. J Urol 1991; 145: 363(A)

26. Astrahan M A, Ameye F, Oyen R et al. Interstitial temperature measurement during transurethral microwave hyperthermia. J Urol 1991; 145: 304–308

27. Lindner A, Braf Z, Lev A et al. Local hyperthermia of the prostate gland for the treatment of benign prostatic hypertrophy and urinary retention. Br J Urol 1990; 65: 201–203

Single-session transurethral microwave thermotherapy: comparison of two therapeutic modes in a multicentre study

4

P. Perrin   M. Devonec   P. Houdelette   P. Colombeau
P. Menguy   M. Peneau   J. Kemper   S. Molhoff   H. Rall
G. Hubmann

Introduction

Four randomized studies have been conducted in Europe[1–4] and in the USA,[5] comparing transurethral microwave thermotherapy (TUMT) with sham treatment of benign prostatic hyperplasia (BPH). They have demonstrated that TUMT brings about a marked improvement of symptoms and a moderate improvement in peak flow.

TUMT has also been randomized to transurethral resection of the prostate (TURP):[6] the two treatment modalities provide a significant improvement in symptoms and peak flow rate (PFR) relative to baseline. The benefit after TUMT and TURP does not differ significantly for symptom score in both groups, but is significantly greater for PFR in the TURP group.

If success is defined as a Madsen symptom score inferior or equal to 3 or a decrease superior or equal to 8 from baseline, and/or a PFR increase of 4 ml/s or a 50% increase from baseline, 70% of patients achieve success after TUMT.[5]

Two studies have been undertaken to characterize a successful outcome after TUMT; the clinical features of patients before treatment were analysed, as well as technical parameters during treatment, as follows.

A *retrospective* clinical study compared responders and non-responders:[7] no significant difference was found between the two groups in relation to clinical parameters before treatment [i.e. age, symptom score, PFR, prostate volume and prostate-specific antigen (PSA)]; however a signficant difference was found between the two groups with regard to treatment parameters (i.e. dose of energy delivered to the prostate, and duration of the period during which urethral temperature is superior to rectal temperature). This study demonstrated that response to TUMT was dose dependent: the higher the energy, the better the results.

In a *prospective* clinical study,[8] interstitial thermometry was performed during treatment and temperature recording was later compared with clinical outcome after TUMT. A significant correlation was found between intraprostatic temperature during treatment and improvement in symptom score as well as PFR at 6 months. The best clinical results were observed in those patients who achieved the highest intraprostatic temperatures.

Consequently, a higher-energy protocol was designed to improve the success rate of TUMT.[9,10] The purpose of this retrospective study was to test the hypothesis 'the higher the energy, the better the results'. The results of two therapeutic regimens were compared: results of higher energy TUMT protocol 2.5 versus results of standard TUMT protocol 2.0. Comparison of the two protocols has shown that the moderate increase in the thermal dose delivered by protocol 2.5 results in a significant improvement in clinical outcome. Unlike treatment protocol 2.0,[11–13] treatment protocol 2.5 can relieve moderate to severe obstruction in BPH.[14]

Patients and methods

The results of two multicentre studies were compared; these were the French multicentre randomized study of sham treatment versus the TUMT protocol 2.0[4] and the European multicentre study, conducted in France and Germany, using the more recent TUMT protocol 2.5. Patient characteristics and results of the TUMT arm (163 patients) treated with protocol 2.0 in the French study were compared with patients and results obtained after protocol 2.5 (72 patients) in the European study. The selection criteria of patients complaining of BPH were the same in the two studies, namely a moderate to severe increase in Madsen symptom score, PFR less than 15 ml/s and postresidual volume (PRV) less than 200 ml.

Treatment protocol 2.5 differs from treatment protocol 2.0 in the following respects: the maximum power output is higher in the former, 70 versus 60 W, respectively; the time between 5 W increments is shorter, 2 versus 3 min; the maximum rectal temperature threshold is higher, 43.5 versus 42.5°C; the maximum energy dose is higher, 219 versus 194 kJ.

Results

Before treatment, comparison of patient characteristics in the two groups (Table 4.1) did not show any signficant difference for age, PRV, prostate volume and PSA. However symptom score [Madsen and American Urological Association (AUA)] and PFR at baseline differed significantly in the two groups: the symptom score in the protocol 2.5 group was significantly higher than that in the protocol 2.0 group, and the PFR of the protocol 2.5 group was significantly lower than that of the protocol 2.0 group. In other words, in the 2.5 group patients were more severely affected than in the 2.0 group.

After treatment, comparison of results at 3 months (Table 4.2) showed significant differences between the two groups, for symptom score and PFR.

Parameter	TUMT treatment protocol*		
	2.0 (n = 163)	2.5 (n = 72)	p
Age (years)	68.2 ± 0.6	66.4 ± 1.0	NS†
Madsen score	14.1 ± 0.3	17.5 ± 0.4	<0.001
AUA score	17.6 ± 0.4	22.6 ± 0.6	<0.001
PFR (ml/s)	10.5 ± 0.2	9.2 ± 0.3	<0.001
PRV (ml)	69 ± 3	77 ± 5	NS

Table 4.1. Characteristics before treatment of patients receiving transurethral microwave thermotherapy (TUMT) according to protocol 2.0 or 2.5

*Values are means±SD; †NS, not significant.

Results for both parameters were significantly better in the 2.5 group than in the 2.0 group.

Treatment side effects were clinically significantly different: the retention rate after protocol 2.5 was 80% compared with 20% after protocol 2.0. A Foley catheter was left in situ for at least 2 weeks after protocol 2.5, compared with 3–7 days after protocol 2.0. Prostatic discomfort was more pronounced and longer (2–4 weeks) after protocol 2.5 than after protocol 2.0 (1 week).

Discussion

Comparison of patient characteristics before treatment did not show any

Parameter	TUMT treatment protocol*		
	2.0 (n = 163)	2.5 (n = 72)	p
Madsen score	14.1	17.5	<0.001
Before 3 months	6.8	6.5	NS†
Change (%)	−48	−62	<0.001
AUA score	17.6	22.6	<0.001
Before 3 months	9.0	8.3	NS
Change (%)	−45	−62	<0.001
PFR (ml/s)	10.5	9.2	<0.001
Before 3 months	12.7	15.2	<0.001
Change (%)	+25	+71	<0.001

Table 4.2. Results at 3 months of TUMT according to treatment protocol 2.0 or 2.5

*Values are means; †NS, not significant.

significant difference between candidates for non-medical treatment of BPH in France and Germany.

Patients selected for the study using the TUMT protocol 2.5 had higher symptom scores and lower PFR scores than patients selected for the study using TUMT protocol 2.0, although the selection criteria were the same in the two studies. Treatment was spontaneously offered to more severely obstructed patients in the study delivering protocol 2.5, probably because the physician was aware of the higher energy protocol and the possibility of a better clinical outcome with that than after protocol 2.0.

The superior results obtained using protocol 2.5 compared with protocol 2.0 relate not only to the percentage change from baseline but also to the absolute figure achieved for symptom score and PFR; indeed, after protocol 2.5, the PFR far exceeds that of patients of the same age but without BPH symptoms (i.e. 13 ml/s at the age of 70 years). After protocol 2.5, the PFR is in the range usually observed after TURP.

Thus this clinical study evaluating a higher-energy TUMT protocol confirmed the hypothesis 'the higher the energy, the better the results'.

The higher-energy protocol is safe, as no severe complication was observed at the level of the upper urinary tract, rectum or striated sphincter. However, side effects were significantly more pronounced than after protocol 2.0, i.e. urinary retention was more frequent and the inflammatory reaction lasted longer. Suprapubic or Foley catheterization for 2–4 weeks following treatment using a new technique is not acceptable. This drawback requires a simple solution; patients should recover satisfactory micturition rapidly, if possible immediately after a day case treatment. The answer probably lies in the use of newer forms of prostatic urethra stenting. Nevertheless, the inflammatory reaction inherent to any modality of heat treatment, such as microwave, laser[15] or focused ultrasound,[16] will remain. In the case of microwave thermotherapy, cooling the urethra throughout the procedure significantly reduces discomfort after TUMT[17,18] when compared with other techniques of heat therapy, which do not spare the urethra. The prescription of non-steroidal anti-inflammatory drugs for 1–2 weeks is mandatory after higher energy protocol 2.5 and helps patients to recover comfortable micturition more rapidly.

In conclusion, the higher-energy protocol 2.5 gives better results than protocol 2.0 but at the price of increased morbidity. The choice between treatment protocol 2.0 or 2.5 should be made according to patient profile: moderate to marked BPH obstruction should preferably be treated using higher-energy TUMT protocol 2.5, whereas mild obstruction should be treated using standard protocol 2.0.

References

1. Perrin P, Devonec M, Fendler JP et al. Thermotherapy versus sham treatment in benign prostatic hypertrophy. Prog Urol 1992; 2(suppl): A50
2. De la Rosette JJMCH, de Wildt MJAM, Alivazatos G et al. Transurethral microwave thermotherapy (TUMT) in benign prostatic hyperplasia: placebo versus TUMT. Urology 1994; in press
3. Ogden CW, Reddy P, Johnson H et al. Sham versus transurethral microwave thermotherapy in patients with symptoms of benign prostatic outflow obstruction. Lancet 1993; 341: 14–17
4. Devonec M, Houdelette P, Colombeau P et al. A multicenter study of sham versus thermotherapy in benign prostatic hypertrophy. J Urol 1994; 151: 415A
5. Blute ML, Patterson DE, Segura JW et al. Transurethral microwave thermotherapy versus sham: a prospective double blind randomized study. J Urol 1994; 151: 415A
6. Dahlstrand C, Geirsson G, Fall M, Pettersson S. Transurethral microwave thermotherapy versus transurethral resection for benign prostatic hyperplasia: preliminary results of a randomized trial. Eur Urol 1993; 23(suppl): 292–298
7. Berg C, Choi N, Colombeau P et al. Responders versus non-responders to thermotherapy in BPH: a multicenter retrospective analysis of a patient and treatment profiles. J Urol 1993; 149: 251A
8. Carter SSTC, Ogden C. Intraprostatic temperature versus clinical outcome in TUMT. Is the response heat-dose dependent? J Urol 1994; 151: 416A
9. Devonec M, Ogden C, Perrin P, Carter SSTC. Clinical response to transurethral microwave thermotherapy is thermal dose dependent. Eur Urol 1993; 23: 267–274
10. Devonec M, Fendler JF, Nasser M et al. The clinical response to transurethral microwave thermotherapy is dose-dependent: from thermo-coagulation to thermo-ablation. J Urol 1993; 149: 249A
11. Rosier PFWM, de Wildt MJAM, Van Kerrebroeck PEVA et al. Urodynamic results of transurethral microwave thermotherapy treatment of 'prostatism'. Neurourol Urodyn 1993; 12: 378–379
12. Höfner K, Tan HK, Kramer AEJL et al. Changes in outflow obstruction in patients with benign prostatic hypertrophy (BPH) after transurethral microwave thermotherapy (TUMT). Neurourol Urodyn 1993; 12: 376–377
13. Tubaro A, Ogden C, De la Rosette JJMCH et al. The prediction of clinical outcome from thermotherapy by pressure-flow study. Results of a European multicenter study. J Urol 1994; 151: 417A
14. De la Rosette J, De Wildt M, Debruyne F. TUMT treatment in patients with BPH: the hotter, the better? Proc 23rd Congr SIU, Sydney, September, 1994: 274.
15. Kabalin JN. Laser prostatectomy performed with a right angle firing neodymium: YAG laser fiber at 40 watts power setting. J Urol 1993; 150: 95–99
16. Madersbacher S, Kratzik C, Szabo N et al. Tissue ablation in benign prostatic hyperplasia with high-intensity focused ultrasound. Eur Urol 1993; 23(suppl 1): 39–43
17. Devonec M, Berger N, Perrin P. Transurethral microwave heating of the prostate: from hyperthermia to thermotherapy. J Endourol 1991; 5: 129–135
18. Cormio L, Bloem F, Laduc R, Debruyne FMJ. Pain sensation in transurethral microwave thermotherapy for benign prostatic hyperplasia: the rationale for prophylactic sedation. Eur Urol 1994; 25: 36–39

Changes in outflow obstruction following transurethral microwave thermotherapy

5

K. Höfner   H. Krah   M. Kuczyk   H. K. Tan
U. Jonas

Introduction

Transurethral microwave thermotherapy (TUMT) is one of the most recent alternative concepts in the treatment of benign prostatic hyperplasia (BPH). This method differs from hyperthermia in that intraprostatic temperatures of 45 and 60°C are achieved.[1]

At the time of writing, 25 000 patients have been treated worldwide in 70 centres with the Prostatron® (Technomed Medical Systems, Lyon, France), with a documented clinical total response rate of 75% (cure in 25% of cases, improvement in 50%, and failure to show any improvement in 25% of cases).

Within the FDA protocol, data obtained during the 18 month follow-up period were made available on over 1000 patients from 16 centres in Europe and in the USA.[2] Improvement of the Madsen symptom score was shown just 4 weeks following TUMT. Objective data, such as increase in peak urinary flow rate (Q_{max}) and reduced residual urine volume, only reached significant levels 3 months after TUMT. The outcome of treatment remained constant up to 18 months in the results published. In double-blind random studies between thermotherapy and sham studies, TUMT gave significantly better results with regard to both subjective and objective data.[3–6] In the random group comparison between TUMT and transurethral resection of the prostate (TURP), improvement of subjective symptoms of patients was statistically identical. Improvement in objective data such as residual urine and maximum urinary flow was statistically considerably lower following TUMT.[7,8] A retrospective multicentre analysis of responders versus non-responders[3,9] revealed that the clinical response rate is dependent on the thermoenergy applied. Meanwhile, alternative software has been developed (Prostasoft 2.5) enabling application of higher levels of energy.

It is still not clear precisely how thermotherapy affects the objective and subjective symptoms of patients with BPH. It is assumed that the subjective symptoms (irritation) are influenced by the evident effect on the autonomic nervous system.[10] A potential effect of thermotherapy on the reduction of outflow resistance may be caused by the shrinkage of tissue due to tissue necrosis, leading to expansion of the urethral lumen in the prostatic urethra.

Urodynamics

Urodynamic pressure flow measurements are the only values suitable for detailed analysis of the extent of change in bladder outflow obstruction (BOO) following therapy of BPH.[1] In almost all studies carried out to test the efficacy of TUMT, the criteria used were subjective symptoms, Q_{max} and residual urine. As no correlation was found between the scores and the degree of outflow obstruction, it was not possible to draw any conclusions about the change of BOO with regard to improvement of subjective symptoms.[11-13] Some problems arise when uroflowmetry, a non-invasive technique, is used as a therapeutic control parameter, as the flow of urine is only the end result of all unknown factors influencing micturition. Additionally, there is a dependence of Q_{max} (the most accepted clinical parameter of uroflowmetry) on the volume voided, rendering it necessary to use nomograms for comparison with normal values. As a result of this dependence of Q_{max} on volume, an increased value of bladder volume due to a specific therapy can generate an increased Q_{max} value without alteration of bladder outlet. On the other hand, a comparison of Q_{max} in different groups is possible only if the differences in voided volumes are not statistically significant. A special index formula is used in the authors' institute.[14] This index is independent of volume and is representative only of other causes of change in Q_{max}. The non-significant value of measured residual urine as an obstruction parameter in BPH patients has been fully documented.[15-19] The only method by which the voiding disturbance caused by the prostate can be assessed objectively is the urodynamic registration of pressure and flow during voiding and its analysis according to well-defined algorithms based on the physical and hydrodynamic properties of bladder and urethra.[20-22] Despite the use of all elements of modern urodynamics, it is still not possible to calculate different specific resistance factors for separate locations within the urethra (internal sphincter, BPH, external sphincter). The interrelationship only of the different channels may be interpreted (i.e. the amount of pressure responsible for each flow)— a very inaccurate procedure. Griffiths[20] introduced the urethral resistance relation (URR; the plot of detrusor pressure versus flow rate) to assess the data objectively. However, because of difficulty in interpretation of complex URR plots, these have not been used routinely for clinical interpretation. Computerized urodynamics enable basic parameters to be extracted from the part of the URR curves that is governed by passive properties of the urethra only, reflecting the minimal resistance exerted by the urethra during voiding (i.e. the hydrodynamic expression of the anatomic mechanical obstruction). The minimal resistance part of the

URR can be seen in the plots as the leg of the curves representing the lowest pressure for each flow rate. A model curve can be fitted to this lowest pressure part, following which the parameters from the model curve can be used to characterize the urethral resistance during voiding. Schäfer[23] idealized his model to a quadratic curve, the passive urethral resistance relation (PURR), using two parameters with clear-cut clinical counterparts—the footpoint (a constant of the model curve: the intersection with the pressure axis, reflecting the urethral opening pressure) and the curvature (gradient, coefficient of the quadratic part of the curve reflecting the area of the flow-controlling zone—the area during flow) (Fig. 5.1).

The urodynamic quantification of the TUMT-induced changes in footpoint and curvature and A_{theo} (a parameter calculated from the PURR curvature,[23] the theoretical cross-sectional area of the flow-controlling zone), respectively, is the most satisfactory method of documenting the objective effect on mechanical outflow obstruction in BPH patients.

Patients and methods

A total of 140 patients with BPH were treated by TUMT (Prostatron®, Prostasoft 2.0, Technomed Medical Systems). Patients with normal clinical indications for treatment of BPH were selected. The main inclusion criteria

Passive Urethral Resistance Relation

p_{det}

Q

p-Q
Plot

p

Flow

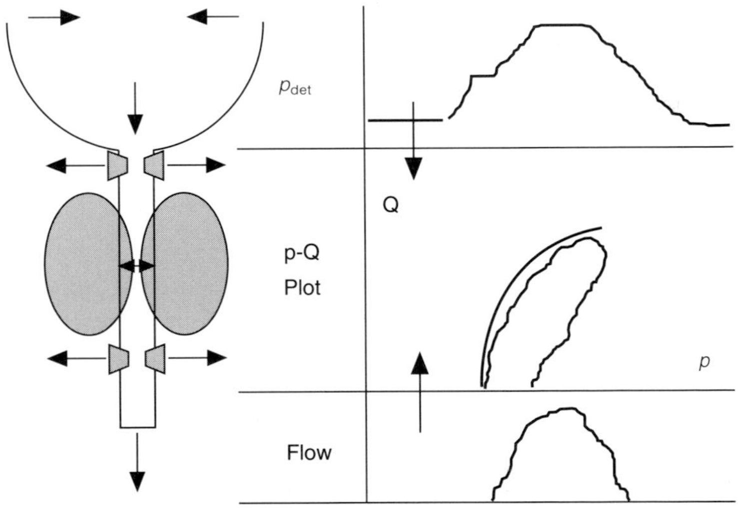

Fig. 5.1. Schematic drawing of passive urethral resistance relation (PURR). By eliminating the time from the pressure (p_{det}) and flow (Q) trends, a two-dimensional p–Q plot results. Each point in this plot represents the pressure and flow values taken from the pressure and flow time trends at the appropriate point in time. The PURR represents the minimal urethral resistance during voiding, caused by the mechanical obstruction component. The footpoint of the PURR (intersection with the pressure axis) represents the urethral opening pressure, its slope the properties of the opened urethra.

were a Madsen symptom score of more than 8, a prostatic urethral length [assessed by transrectal ultrasound (TRUS)] of 35–50 mm, a Q_{max} value of less than 15 ml/s with voided volume of more than 150 ml, and no evidence of prominent prostatic middle lobe or bladder neck sclerosis. Patients with suspected prostatic carcinoma and patients with neurogenic voiding dysfunction were not included in this study. Treatment could not be carried out in two patient owing to failure to introduce the transurethral heating catheter, and in three patients the treatment had to be discontinued owing to pain during application. Follow-ups were scheduled at 1 and 6 weeks, 3 and 6 months and 1 year after treatment. Before treatment and at each follow-up, Madsen scores and a voiding diary were taken and urine flow rate and prostatic volume (by TRUS) were estimated. Cystometry and pressure/flow studies were performed before treatment and at the 3 month follow-up. The computerized urodynamic set-up [AUDIT™ (Advanced Urodynamic Data Interpretation Technology), FM Wiest][24–26] analysed the pressure/flow data according to the PURR in the footpoint and curvature and calculated the obstruction parameter as well as the contractility parameter (W).[27] All these parameters and various other patient data scores, free flow and cystometry were compared with regard to findings before and after treatment, with paired t tests. The significance level was set at 0.05.

As 24 patients declined to take part in the follow-up schedule, they were treated without pretreatment urodynamic assessment. Drop-outs from the study occurred at 1 week (3 of 104 patients), 6 weeks (7 of 92—one with transurethral resection), 3 months (2 of 78—one with transurethral resection), 6 months (8 of 62) and 12 months (1 of 19). Of the 71 patients with pretreatment urodynamic assessment, 32 have now passed the 3 month follow-up with urodynamic assessment.

Results

As shown in Table 5.1, and in accordance with the results of international studies, the symptom score showed rapid improvement, with regard to obstructive as well as irritative symptoms. The urinary outflow rate showed a significant increase, even following volume correction (flow index[14]). No significant changes occurred in urethral opening pressure, URR or PURR footpoint. In contrast to the experiences of other centres, the changes in residual urine volume were non-significant. Objective data obtained from cystometry (maximum bladder capacity, first sensation) were unchanged. Prostate volume measured by TRUS showed a significant decrease of about 16%.

The calculated value only of the theoretical cross-sectional area during flow (A_{theo}) (Fig. 5.2) showed a significant increase after treatment. The detrusor contractility was not influenced. The increase of the PURR

Urodynamic parameter	Before treatment (n=32)	At 3 month follow-up (n=32)	Significance of change (p)
Obstruction score	9.94	3.12	0.000
Irritation score	5.36	3.63	0.017
Q_{max}** (ml/s)	11.29	15.08	0.003
Flow index	2.69	3.31	0.011
Residual urine (ml)	92.3	95.1	0.884
BPH volume (cm^3)	35.7	30.0	0.003
Opening pressure (cmH_2O)	64.2	67.9	0.567
PURR† footpoint (cmH_2O)	54.0	52.6	0.820
A_{theo}† (mm^2)	3.11	5.26	0.018
W_{max}‡ (W/m^2)	14.4	13.2	0.676

Table 5.1. Results* of urodynamic assessment of patients with benign prostatic hyperplasia (BPH) treated by transurethral microwave thermotherapy (TUMT)

*Values are means; **Q_{max}, peak urinary flow rate; †for explanation of PURR and A_{theo} see text; ‡W_{max}, peak value of contractility during voiding.

curvature on an unchanged footpoint corresponds to an improvement in the elasticity of the prostatic urethra, which was reported in all results in which there was improvement of urine flow (Fig. 5.3).

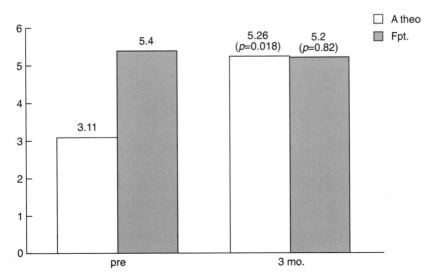

Fig. 5.2. Changes of PURR footpoint (■) and cross-sectional area of the flow-controlling zone (A_{theo}; □) after transurethral microwave thermotherapy (TUMT). pre, before treatment; 3 mo., at 3 month follow-up.

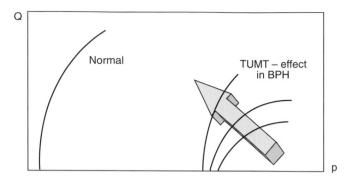

Fig. 5.3. TUMT effect in BPH: increased steepness of the PURR without alteration of the PURR footpoint, resulting in flow improvement.

Discussion

This study investigated to what extent TUMT, a non-ablative procedure, is able to reduce the outflow resistance brought about by possible shrinkage of the intraprostatic BPH tissue. Although an improvement has been confirmed in the literature regarding subjective symptoms and Q_{max} in urine flow, other than the theoretical cross-sectional area of the flow-controlling zone (A_{theo}), no changes were recorded in the classic parameter of the pressure/flow measurements. In this respect, one cannot compare results of TUMT and TURP when analysed in relation to the documented effect of TURP on the reduction of mechanical outflow resistance. This is not surprising, considering that the non-ablative procedure of TUMT is being compared with tissue resection with TURP. Furthermore, TUMT exerts a specific effect on outflow obstruction that cannot be compared quantitatively with TURP. On opening of the urethra during micturition following TUMT, it is essential that a urethral opening pressure identical to that before treatment is achieved. The improvement in the elasticity of the prostatic urethra brought about by TUMT results in a significant reduction of the pressure necessary following opening of the urethra during micturition. The data regarding objective changes of outflow obstruction have meanwhile been confirmed internationally in retrospective analyses on responders/non-responders, indicating that the TUMT responders, in particular, display a compressive type of obstruction (flat PURR curve).[28,29]

The effects of the new alternative method of treatment should be appraised with caution. This applies to all forms of BPH therapy, including the 'Gold standard' TURP which, after 40 years, has demonstrated clearly the success rate and complications involved in such a procedure.

In the USA, 400 000 patients per year undergo transurethral prostatectomy. TURP is the most frequently performed operation on the urogenital tract and is the second most expensive surgical procedure, for which US$5 $\times 10^9$ are paid out yearly.[30] The general response rate lies at 80%, the mortality rate has decreased to 1% over the past 20 years and the morbidity rate remains unchanged at 18%.[31,32] TURP can only be performed under anaesthesia on an inpatient basis. Blood transfusions are necessary in 6.5–10%. Postoperative complications include impotence (3.5–10%), incontinence (0.4–2.3%), urinary tract infection (2.3–8.4%), epididymitis (1.2–4.8%), a longer catheterization period (8.7–21.2% on day 5 after operation), urethral strictures (3.5%) and bladder neck sclerosis (3%); retrograde ejaculation is experienced by the majority of patients.[31–33] In 15% of patients a second TURP procedure is required within a period of 10 years.[34]

The complications involved in TURP will have to be accepted until more effective treatment becomes available. In view of the increasing number of alternative concepts, the different outcomes of alternative procedures and TURP warrant investigation. In the study carrried out by Dahlstrand et al,[35] TUMT has been compared with TURP and it has been shown that improvement in objective data such as maximal urinary flow rate and residual urine can not be achieved in the same way as with TURP. Improvement in subjective symptoms is comparable to that found after TURP. Complications arising in TUMT are considerably less than those with TURP, with regard to the mortality and morbidity rates. The known complications of TURP, such as impotence, retrograde ejaculation, intraoperative and postoperative bleeding requiring therapy, urethral strictures and urinary incontinence do not occur following thermotherapy. TUMT can be performed on an outpatient basis and without anaesthesia. Some patients, however, require an antispasmodic analgesic during the course of treatment. An effective reduction of outflow resistance as shown by pressure/flow measurements has been documented for TURP,[35–38] indicating the efficacy of the TURP procedure in the elimination of specific mechanical obstruction in BPH. This fact indicates that TURP is effective because of the tissue ablation involved. Retrospective studies have revealed, however, that 30% of those patients treated by TURP do not have any obstruction, which suggests that this group of patients may derive just as much benefit from a minimally invasive procedure that dispenses with the need for tissue ablation and has only a minimal effect on obstruction. TUMT (Prostasoft 2.0) cannot be compared with an ablative procedure such as transurethral resection. This refers to the effect on outflow obstruction as well as the considerably lower rate of complications. As TUMT is comparable to TURP with regard to improvement of subjective symptoms, however, the outflow obstruction is not significantly changed. TUMT would prove, therefore, an optimal choice for BPH patients with a low-grade obstruction. As opposed to drug therapy, TUMT has the advantage in that it is performed once only. Minimal obstructive BPH does not necessarily have to progress to the more serious stage before TUMT may be performed, making the latter an ideal form of therapy for BPH patients.

In cases involving minimal urodynamic obstruction, TURP may not be justified, because of the higher rate of complications and the lack of necessity for surgical resection. Transurethral resection of the prostate continues to be carried out for BPH with mechanical obstruction. Here, transurethral resection of the prostate is competing with other ablative procedures, such as laser treatment. It remains to be seen to what extent an increase in energy with TUMT (intraprostatic temperature increased to 70°C) will result in an ablation of prostate tissue ('thermoablation') using the available software Prostasoft 2.5. It is imperative that clinical studies are carried out to assess objectively this form of therapy for obstructive BPH.

References

1. Smith P H, Marberger M, Conort P et al. Other non-medical therapies (excluding lasers) in the treatment of BPH. Proc 2nd Inter Consultation Benign Prostatic Hyperplasia (BPH) Paris, 27–30 June, 1993: 453–491
2. Laduc R, Bloem F A G, Debruyne F M J. Transurethral microwave thermotherapy in symptomatic benign prostatic hyperplasia. Eur Urol 1993; 23: 275–281
3. Devonec M, Ogden C, Perrin P, Carter S St C. Clinical response to transurethral microwave thermotherapy is thermal dose dependent. Eur Urol 1993; 23: 267–274
4. Ogden C, Johnson H, Patel A et al. A single prospective study of SHAM versus TUMT in symptomatic prostatic bladder outflow obstruction, initial results. In: Giuliani L, Puppo P (eds) Urology. Bologna: Monduzzi Editore, 1992: 247–250
5. Ogden C W, Reddy P, Johnson H et al. Sham versus transurethral microwave thermotherapy in patients with symptoms of benign prostatic bladder outflow obstruction. Lancet 1993; 341: 14–17
6. Blute M L, Patterson D E, Segura J W et al. Transurethral microwave thermotherapy versus sham treatment. A randomized double blind study. J Endourol 1993; 7(suppl 1): S124
7. Dahlstrand C, Geirsson G, Fall M, Petterson S. Transurethral microwave thermotherapy versus transurethral resection for benign prostatic hyperplasia: preliminary results of a randomized study. Eur Urol 1993; 23: 292–298
8. Pettersson S, Dahlstrand C, Fall M, Giersson G. Transurethral microwave thermotherapy versus transurethral resection for benign prostatic hyperplasia: preliminary results of a randomized study. J Urol 1992; 147: 305A
9. Devonec M, Fendler J P, Joubert P et al. Responders versus non responders to thermotherapy in BPH: a multicentre analysis of patients and treatment profiles (230 cases). J Endourol 1993; 7(suppl 1): S77
10. Perachino M, Bozzo W, Puppo P et al. Does transurethral thermotherapy induce a long-term alpha blockade? Eur Urol 1993; 23: 299–301
11. Barry M J, Cockett A T K, Holtgrewe H L et al. Relationship of symptoms of prostatism to commonly used physiological and anatomical measures of the severity of benign prostatic hyperplasia. J Urol 1993; 150: 351–358
12. Chapple C R. Correlation of symptomatology, urodynamics, morphology and size of the prostate in benign prostatic hyperplasia. Curr Opinion Urol 1993; 3: 5–9
13. Rosier P, Rollema H J, van de Beek C, Janknegt R A. Are symptoms reliable guides in assessing the pathologic condition of the lower urinary tract? J Urol 1992; 147: 367A
14. Höfner K, Kramer A E J L, Allhoff E P, Jonas U. A new uroflow-index—clinical experience. J Urol 1992; 140: 269A
15. Anderson J B, Grant J B. Postoperative retention of urine: a prospective urodynamic study. Br Med J 1991; 302: 894–896
16. Jensen K M-E, Jorgensen J B, Mogensen P. Urodynamics in prostatism. III. Prognostic value of medium-fill water cystometry. Scand J Urol Nephrol 1988; 114(suppl): 78–83

17. Robertson A S, Airey R, Griffiths C J et al. Detrusor contraction strength in men undergoing prostatectomy. Neurourol Urodyn 1993; 12: 109–121
18. Tan H K, Höfner K, Kramer A E J L et al. Benign prostatic hypertrophy (BPH): prostatic size, obstruction parameters, detrusor contractility and their independence. Neurourol Urodyn 1993; 12: 412–413
19. Van Mastrigt R, Rollema H J. The prognostic value of bladder contractility in transurethral resection of the prostate. J Urol 1992; 148: 1856–1860
20. Griffiths D J. Urodynamics. The mechanics and hydrodynamics of the lower urinary tract. Medical Physics Handbooks 4. Bristol: Adam Higler, 1980
21. Schäfer W. The contribution of the bladder outlet to the relation between pressure and flow rate during micturition. In: Hinman F Jr (ed) Benign prostatic hypertrophy. New York: Springer Verlag, 1983; 470–496
22. Spångberg A, Teriö H, Engberg A, Ask P. Quantification of urethral function based on Griffiths' model of flow through elastic tubes. Neurourol Urodyn 1989; 8: 29–52
23. Schäfer W. Urethral resistance? Urodynamic concepts of physiological and pathological bladder outlet function during voiding. Neurourol Urodyn 1985; 4: 161–201
24. Höfner K, Meßtechnik in der Urodynamik—Standortbestimmung, Trends und eigenes Konzept. In: Jonas U (ed) Jahrbuch der Urologie 1992. Zülpich: Biermann-Verlag, 1992; 31–43
25. Höfner K. Urodynamic evaluation of lower urinary tract dysfunction. Curr Opinion Urol 1992; 2: 257–262
26. Höfner K, Börner K, Schäfer W et al. Advanced Urodynamic Data Intepretation Technology (AUDIT^{TM})—a new software for urodynamic investigations. J Urol 1993; 149: 236A
27. Griffiths D, van Mastrigt R, Bosch R. Quantification of urethral resistance and bladder function during voiding, with special reference to the effects of prostate size reduction on urethral obstruction due to benign prostatic hyperplasia. Neurourol Urodyn 1989; 8: 17–27
28. Dahlstrand C, Geirsson G, Waldén W et al. Can pressure flow measurement and obstruction grading predict outcome after TUR-P or TUMT? J Endourol 1993; 7(suppl 1): S77
29. Trucchi A, Tubaro A, Galatioto G P et al. Responders versus non-responders to transurethral microwave thermotherapy. A retrospective analysis. J Endourol 1993; 7(suppl 1): S77
30. Holtgrewe H L, Mebust W K, Dowd J B. Transurethral prostadectomy: practice aspects of the dominant operation in American urology. J Urol 1989; 141: 248–253
31. Mebust W K, Holtgrewe H I, Cockett A T K et al. Transurethral prostatectomy: immediate and prospective complications. A cooperative study of 13 participating institutions evaluating 3,885 patients. J Urol 11989; 141: 243
32. Melchior J, Valk W L, Foret J D, Mebust W K. Transurethral prostatectomy: computerized analysis of 2,233 cases. J Urol 1974; 112: 634–642
33. Mebust W K. Surgical management of benign prostatic obstruction. Urology 1991: 32(suppl 6): 12–15
34. Wennberg J E, Roos N, Sola L et al. Use of claims data system to evaluate health care outcomes. Mortality and reoperation after prostatectomy. JAMA 1987; 257
35. Dahlstrand C, Geirsson G, Fall M, Petterson S. Transurethral microwave thermotherapy versus transurethral resection for benign prostatic hyperplasia: preliminary results of a randomized study. Eur Urol 1993; 23: 292–298
36. Schäfer W, Noppeney R, Rübben H, Lutzeyer W. The value of free flow rate and pressure flow studies in the routine investigation of BPH-patients. Neurourol Urodyn 1989; 7: 219–221
37. Van Mastrigt R, Rollema H J. Urethral resistance and urinary bladder contractility before and after transurethral resection as determined by the computer program CLIM. Neurourol Urodyn 1988; 7: 226–228
38. Schäfer W, Rübben H, Noppeney R, Deutz F J. Obstructed and unobstructed prostatic obstruction. World J Urol 1989; 6: 198–203

Thermal dose calculations in the treatment of symptomatic prostatism with high-temperature microwave thermotherapy

6

J. Trachtenberg   A. Toi   E. Yeung   F. Habib

Introduction

The treatment of benign prostatic hyperplasia (BPH) is currently evolving from the traditional approach of watchful waiting, followed by surgery when warranted, to a myriad of less invasive alternatives. The last decade has seen an enormous amount of effort devoted to offering innovative options to patients with symptomatic BPH. The stimulus for these efforts is to try to duplicate the excellent results of surgery but to eliminate the known complications of treatment and to do so in an outpatient setting in a cost-effective manner. New options have included several novel pharmacological approaches, such as the use of alpha-adrenergic blocking agents to decrease the tone of intraprostatic smooth muscle; as well as five alpha-reductase inhibitors that decrease prostatic bulk and in turn decrease prostatic urethral resistance.[1,2] Several new surgical techniques have also been described recently; these include laser ablation of the prostate as well as various means of heating the prostate to decrease symptoms.[3,4] One of the most explored forms of heat-induced therapy of the prostate uses microwave energy.[5]

Early research into the use of microwaves to treat BPH sought to achieve temperatures that were higher than body temperature but lower than 45°C, and is termed 'hyperthermia'. Treatments were performed with both transurethral and transrectal applicators and usually required multiple treatment sessions. Treatments in this range did not create any histological changes in prostatic tissue and demonstrated questionable improvement in objective parameters; most clinical effects were not sustained.

Owing in large measure to the pioneering efforts of Marian Devonec, microwave thermotherapy of the prostate has become a more understood treatment option for BPH.[5] Thermotherapy attempts to subject the target tissue to a sustained temperature above 45°C, which should cause irreversible damage to the prostate. None the less, the results of many trials are often contradictory. Although attaining a temperature 'above

45°C' appeared to deliver better results than one 'below 45°C', researchers often failed to show any histological or structural change to prostatic tissue.[6] Possible explanations for this might be that the temperature sought after might not have been reached, or, if reached, was not sustained for long enough. Few researchers monitored the temperature within the prostate on each of the patients studied, to document whether target temperatures were reached, or if reached, for how long that target temperature was sustained.

More recently, however, it has been suggested that treating the gland with microwaves at higher temperatures (up to 70°C) would more definitively destroy tissue and that the therapy that would result would have longer-lasting effects. It has also been suggested that the results are dose dependent. Although the target temperature was identified by these researchers, the temperatures achieved and the location of these high temperatures within the prostate were never reported. Lastly, an apparent disadvantage of the goal to achieve very high target temperatures is the necessity of administering general anaesthesia. This development shifts the setting of care from an office or outpatient-orientated treatment towards an inpatient treatment, defeating one of the main advantages of this new form of therapy. The authors have explored the use of transurethral microwave thermotherapy of the prostate to determine the optimal use and effectiveness of this mode of treatment.

Patients and methods

In view of the apparent benefits of achieving higher intraprostatic temperatures, described above, it was the technical and clinical goal of this study to develop a microwave system that would enable higher (above 55°C) temperatures to be achieved within the prostate without the need for general anaesthesia. In addition, intraprostatic temperatures were measured at a particular and repeatable place in the gland of each patient to gain a better understanding of the pathophysiology of microwave-induced thermal damage to the prostate.

Sixty-two patients aged 55–80 years, with symptomatic BPH who wanted treatment were enrolled in an experimental protocol to assess the safety and effectiveness of a second-generation prostatic thermotherapy device (UroWave, Dornier Medical Systems, Inc., Kennesaw, GA, USA). All patients signed an informed consent form before embarking on this trial. All patients had a diagnosis of symptomatic BPH confirmed by rectal examination and transrectal ultrasound. All patients had an American Urological Association (AUA) symptom score of greater than 15 and a peak urinary flow rate of less than 12 ml/s. No patient had any prior medical or surgical treatment for prostatism. Patients with pacemakers or metallic prostheses in their pelvis were excluded. Patients with a suspicion of prostate or bladder cancer, neurogenic bladder, history of urinary retention, or impaired upper tracts were also excluded. No patient was taking any medication known to affect voiding function. Patients with a large obstructing middle lobe of the prostate, as noted at cystoscopy, were also excluded.

All treatments were administered as outpatient therapy, without provision for general anaesthesia. The Urowave applies 915 MHz microwave energy to the prostate via a helical coil antenna enclosed in a transurethral delivery system. Some existing transurethral microwave delivery systems have attempted to cool the delivery system, both to preserve the urethra and, perhaps more importantly, to help minimize pain when trying to deliver higher temperatures.[7] Careful examination of the design of these delivery systems reveals, however, that only about one-half of the urethra is being cooled and that hot spots can easily occur. Furthermore, the catheter wall thickness separating the cooling water from the prostatic urethra is such that the cooling of that part of the urethra that is cooled, is very inefficient, because of the insulation provided by the catheter wall. The design of the delivery system used in this study provides for some important improvements over current designs. The antenna is enclosed inside an inner lumen of a catheter through which water cooling is provided. Surrounding this inner catheter is a very thin (0.015 mm) non-distensible membrane. Cooling water is pressurized and flows through the inner catheter into the inside of the outer balloon, inflating it to 18 Fr to provide intimate contact with the mucosa of the urethra. The thin membrane is efficient in terms of removing heat from the urethral mucosa and provides 360 degrees of uninterrupted cooling of the entire urethral mucosa. When collapsed, prior to insertion, the catheter is only 9 Fr, making insertion easier and more comfortable for the patient than the traditional 20 Fr or larger catheters used in other systems.

Power was incrementally increased by a computer-driven algorithm that minimized patient discomfort while raising intraprostatic temperature. The urethral temperature was constantly monitored by an optical thermosensor applied to the outer wall of the cooling balloon that surrounded the antenna. Power was stopped if the urethral temperature exceeded 44.5°C. Similarly, a rectal sensor ensured that rectal temperature never exceeded 42.5°C. Intraprostatic temperatures were measured at eight sites by optical thermosensors. The sensors were housed in two fibre-optic bundles (four sensors each side) and were introduced transperineally under transrectal ultrasound guidance. One four-sensor array was placed to the right and one to the left, 1 cm lateral and parallel to the urethra. Temperature was recorded real time from all sensors but the highest temperature recorded at any site was used as the reference temperature on which treatment was based. Patients were subjected to a 60 min treatment in an outpatient setting. Pain and anxiety were managed with intravenous diazepam when necessary. General or neuroleptic anaesthesia was never used. All measurements were viewed real time on a video display monitor and recorded on disk for later analysis. At the end of the procedure all patients were discharged home with a small indwelling urethral catheter for 3–4 days; during this period patients received oral broad-spectrum antibiotics. After treatment, patients were followed according to the FDA guidance document issued to assess the safety and effectiveness of various alternative treatments for symptomatic BPH.

Results

Intraprostatic temperatures

In most patients, a consistent pattern of prostatic heating emerged from the treatments (Fig. 6.1). During initial heating of the prostate, the thermosensors recorded a slow and steady increase of temperature over the initial 6–10 min, during which time the microwave power delivered increased steadily to its maximum of 80 W. Temperature increased by an average of 1.22 ± 0.13 (mean $\pm$ SEM)°C/min (range 0.85–1.60°C/min).

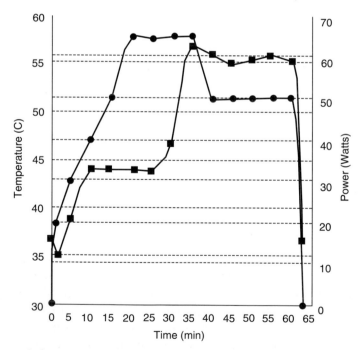

Fig. 6.1. Applied microwave power (–●–) and resulting intraprostatic temperature (–■–) in a patient receiving prostatic thermotherapy treatment. Temperature sensor array was 1 cm lateral and parallel to the urethra. The temperature noted was the highest of a single sensor.

Following this 'slow initial' phase of heating, although power was at its maximum, a 'plateau' phase was noted, which was characterized by a lack of appreciable increase in temperature. The average rate of increase of this phase was only $0.13 \pm 0.07°C/min$. The duration of the plateau was variable (range 7–35 min). However, during the 'post-plateau' heating phase there was a rapid rise of temperature ($3.3 \pm 1.1°C/min$). Microwave power was adjusted (lowered) to achieve the specific target temperature. This phase of heating required close attention with a decrease in power 4–5°C below the desired temperature to prevent an 'overshoot'. The 'post-plateau' phase of treatment always required less power than the power used to reach the plateau phase.

Rectal and urethral temperatures were often stable and below the prescribed limits (44.5°C, urethral; 42.5°C, rectal) even when high intraprostatic temperatures were being achieved. Conversely, patient discomfort seemed capable of triggering a power shut-off when rectal temperatures reached 42.5°C, even if intraprostatic temperatures were low (often less than 45°C). This was felt to be due to the patient clamping down on the rectal probe and pressing it firmly into the prostate. Patient instruction and proper repositioning of the rectal probe usually lowered the temperature reading below the trip limit and the treatment could proceed. There was no correlation between urethral or rectal temperature and intraprostatic temperature.

Thermal dose calculations were performed by multiplying the continuously measured intraprostatic temperature over 45°C (in degrees centigrade) by the time (in seconds) for which the temperature was maintained ($°C \times s$).

Clinical outcome

Side effects

Side effects of treatment were minimal and usually reversible in the 62 patients treated. No patient was hospitalized for any complication. The most common complaint was of discomfort during the procedure. In 82% of patients, either gross or microscopic haematuria was noted. Gross haematuria was usually intermittent, and stopped in all patients by 6 weeks. No patient required a transfusion. No patient became incontinent. Two patients noted lack of ejaculation. It is of interest that semen was not found in the urine, suggesting a sclerotic change to the prostatic and ejaculatory ducts as opposed to damage to the bladder neck. No patient noted any change in potency. Three patients required recatheterization after the initial removal of the catheter. All resumed normal voiding by a maximum of 14 days. No infectious complications were noted.

Clinical results

A total of 52 patients have now been evaluated for at least 12 months. The clinical parameters of change in peak flow rate, as well as changes in International Prostate Symptom Score (IPSS) that were observed are shown in Table 6.1. These values were measured at 1, 3 and 6 months and 1 year. At 12 months, mean peak urine flow rates (Q_{max}) had increased 40% and symptom scores had declined by 50%. Almost three-quarters of patients were clinically improved (as defined by a greater than 33% decrease in symptom scores). In addition, at 6 and 12 months cystoscopic evaluations were performed. The presence of a prostatic fossa defect was noted in 94% of the patients at 12 months. It is noteworthy that, although a prostatic cavity was evident, the bladder neck appeared to be unaffected in most subjects.

Clinical response was also assessed by thermal dose measurements. When patients were arbitrarily divided into groups receiving either less or more than $50\,000°C \times s$, significant differences in Q_{max} were noted between the groups. The 12 month mean increase in Q_{max} in the lower thermal dose range was only 11%, whereas the higher thermal dose group had a mean increase of 48% (Table 6.2). However, symptom scores showed no significant differences between the groups at 6 months (49 and 46% decrease, respectively) or 12 months (Table 6.2).

A responder analysis was also performed. Patients were arbitrarily divided into groups with a Q_{max} increase of less than 30%, more than 30%, and more than 50%. The mean thermal dose for these three increasingly effective treatments was $85\,000°C \times s$, $96\,000°C \times s$, and $111\,000°C \times s$, respectively. The mean 12 month percentage increase in Q_{max} was 2.4, 81 and 93% for these three groups, respectively (Table 6.3a). Interestingly, as in the thermal dose responses, symptom scores did not show major differences in these three Q_{max} responder groups (Table 6.3b).

Parameter†	Assessment time (months)					
	0 (baseline)	1	3	6	9	12
IPSS	22.6±0.6	16.3±0.8	10.8±0.8	11.4±1.0	12.2±1.0	11.2±0.8
%Improved	—	47	82	72	67	71
Q_{max}	8.3±0.6	11±0.7	11.3±1.0	11.5±0.6	11.8±0.7	11.6±0.6
TUR defect	0	—	—	92%	—	94%

Table 6.1. Clinical results* of thermotherapy of BPH with the Urowave

*n=52 patients at 12 months.
†IPSS, International Prostate Symptom Score (±SEM); %Improved, percentage of patients with >33% decrease in IPSS symptom score, Q_{max}, peak urinary flow rate (ml/s±SEM; voided volume >150 ml); TUR defect, percentage of patients with a cystoscopically evident transurethral resection (TUR)-like defect.

Parameter† TD‡		Assessment time (months)				
		1	3	6	9	12
Q_{max}	<50 000	24	20	16	20	11
	>50 000	39	43	47	46	48
IPSS	<50 000	−30	−41	−49	−42	−39
	>50 000	−26	−57	−46	−48	−51

Table 6.2. Mean percentage change over baseline by thermal dose group*

*n=52 patients at 12 months.
†IPSS, International Prostate Symptom Score (percentage change over baseline); Q_{max}, peak urinary flow rate (ml/s; voided volume >150 ml, percentage change over baseline).
‡TD, thermal dose (°C × s).

Symptomatic responses generally improved over the first 3 months. However, patients who were treated at higher temperatures had a slower rate of improvement of symptoms in these first months and took longer to achieve a beneficial effect. Presumably, this was because they received higher temperature treatments that destroyed more prostatic tissue, and a larger tissue response was triggered. Cystoscopic examination of patients treated at high temperatures, even with good clinical results, often showed incomplete healing of the prostatic fossa at 6 months. Because one must wait for the prostate to slough or to be resorbed, or for shrinkage of

(a) In Q_{max}

Group*	Assessment time (months)				
	1	3	6	9	12
1	16	16	9	9	2.4
2	75	73	76	81	81
3	69	81	82	92	93

(b) In AUA symptom score

Group*	Assessment time (months)				
	1	3	6	9	12
1	−31	−52	−44	−42	−46
2	−27	−50	−48	−48	−46
3	−25	−52	−51	−57	−58

Table 6.3. Mean percentage change over baseline by responder group

*Group 1=Q_{max} <30% increase over baseline, mean thermal dose=85 000; group 2=Q_{max} >30% increase over baseline, mean thermal dose=96 000; group 3=Q_{max} >50% increase over baseline, mean thermal dose=110 000.

coagulated tissue to take place, long follow-up times of at least 1 year are probably necessary to assess definitively the outcomes from the different thermal doses and peak temperatures achieved.

Discussion

This is the largest study reported to date in which actual intraprostatic temperatures have been measured in patients during thermotherapy for BPH. One of the most important conclusions from this study is that high intraprostatic temperatures can be achieved in patients without general anaesthesia. This treatment leads to a defect in the prostatic fossa similar to that seen with transurethral resection of the prostate (TURP). These observations pose certain questions.

Although thermotherapy of the prostate is widely practised throughout the world, there are legitimate doubts concerning the reproducibility of the technique. There are two possible explanations for this.

First, target temperature probably needs to be higher than 45°C and needs to be sustained for a defined period over the obstructing tissue. As most investigators do not know what peak temperature has been achieved (because it has not been measured) nor where the temperature was elevated, it is understandable why results are not uniform. Reproducible therapeutic effects require reaching a sufficiently high intraprostatic temperature for a predetermined period over a significant portion of the obstructing prostatic tissue. Critical parameters (peak and duration of intraprostatic temperature rise, site and extent of thermal injury) need to be further defined and standardized such that the technique and results can be duplicated by different investigators and with different devices. Methods to assess thermal dose and monitor it during the therapy appear to be necessary and are part of the authors' effort to optimize this technique. In their opinion, the preliminary thermal dose analysis used in this trial should give greater ability to treat reproducibly and effectively. On-line sonographic imaging with computer enhancement or magnetic resonance imaging of the prostate during treatment to visualize the path of thermal injury may help in this regard. Until these devices are available, direct temperature measurements of intraprostatic temperature will be necessary.

Second, the pathophysiology of the thermal insult to the prostate must be more carefully elucidated and exploited. The biphasic response of the prostate to heating that was observed appears to be a result of the gland's attempt to thermoregulate itself. The 'plateau phase' in Fig. 6.1 illustrates the ability of the prostate gland to maintain an almost constant temperature while being exposed to increasing amounts of heat. The authors consider that this is due to marked vasodilation of the gland and a 'shunting' away of excess heat from the prostate. The duration of this period probably reflects the tissue composition and vascularity of the gland.

As this composition is known to vary markedly in different individuals, it is not surprising that the duration of the plateau phase differs in most patients. It is likely that the 'post-plateau' phase, in which there is a rapid rise in the rate of heating, is due to vascular collapse, probably associated with coagulation of part of the blood supply. Temperature can be maintained in this phase at a markedly reduced microwave power level. The rapid rate of rise of temperature in this latter phase resembles earlier experiments in vitro performed with an avascular phantom model of the prostate. Indeed, the observation of decreased blood flow in this period suggests that part of the vascular supply to the gland has been damaged.

No external parameter of heating, applied wattage, or urethral or rectal temperature correlated with the actual intraprostatic temperature or ultimate tissue destruction. This observation further suggests that a uniform result of treatment can be obtained only if the temperature within the prostate and the extent of thermal injury are known at the time of treatment, to guide the therapy.

The clinical results of this trial are preliminary; furthermore, this trial is single armed, unblinded and not controlled. None the less, sustained improvement in both objective and subjective measures in most of the patients has been shown. This treatment has produced a TURP-like defect in most of the patients, while preserving the bladder neck. These results cannot be accounted for by the well-known placebo effects seen in the treatment of BPH. This has been accomplished in a single-session outpatient setting without the use of general anaesthesia. The side effects are minimal. This is in contrast to the results of Corcos et al,[6] using a device where intraprostatic temperatures were not available on line (the Prostatron), flow rate changes were not maintained and no tissue damage was noted at 6 months. Furthermore, thermal dose analysis of the results in this trial demonstrates that higher sustained temperatures within the prostate are more likely to achieve beneficial results. Conversely, a low thermal dose delivered to the prostate is unlikely to achieve the desired changes in Q_{max}. These results may also suggest that very high temperatures in the prostate may not always be necessary: slightly lower temperatures (over the thermotherapy threshold) for prolonged durations may be as effective as high temperature for shorter durations. This observation has important implications for patient comfort, effectiveness of treatment in patients unable to tolerate very high temperatures, and for patient throughput.

Although the results obtained with the Urowave are clearly not as good as those obtained by conventional surgery, most patients expressed satisfaction with the outcome. These results are similar to, or better than, those reported with other thermotherapy or laser devices at 1 year and better than most pharmacological manipulations.[6,7] It is of interest that cystoscopic inspection of the prostatic fossa showed incomplete healing in some patients even after 12 months of follow-up; this may suggest continuing improvement in the clinical results.

As a defect in the prostatic fossa similar to that with TURP did not increase flow rates to the same extent as TURP, attention should probably be turned to the influence of the bladder neck in the development of outflow obstruction. Indeed, patients with high thermal doses delivered to the prostate and excellent responses need to be assessed to see whether thermal injury to this structure has occurred in spite of normal cystoscopic appearance. More careful urodynamic evaluation of the bladder neck may allow for a more deliberate and planned ablative procedure (ablation of the prostate with or without the bladder neck). Minor ablation of the bladder neck with a planned and thorough injury to the prostate itself may allow the goal of these forms of therapy to be realized, namely safe outpatient single-session treatment without anaesthesia, with minimal morbidity and results comparable to those of surgery.

Acknowledgements

Portions of this paper were read at the Annual meeting of the American Urological Association (San Francisco, May 1994) and have been accepted for publication in the Canadian Journal of Urology.

This study was funded by Dornier Medical Systems, Atlanta, GA, USA.

References

1. Finasteride Study Group. Finasteride (MK 906) in the treatment of benign prostatic hyperplasia. Prostate 1993; 22: 291–299
2. Lepor H. Non operative management of benign prostatic hyperplasia. J Urol 1989; 141: 1183
3. Roth, R A, Babayan R, Aretz H T. TULIP–transurethral ultrasound guided laser induced prostatectomy. J Urol 1991; 145(2): 390a (abstr 712)
4. Norris J P, Norris D M, Lee R D, Rubenstein M A. Visual laser ablation of the prostate: clinical experience in 108 patients. J Urol 1993; 150: 1612–1614
5. Devonec M, Berger N, Perrin P. Transurethral microwave heating of the prostate—or from hyperthermia to thermotherapy. J Endourol 1991; 5: 129
6. Corcos J, Elewedy S, Selemy G, Elhilali M M. Urodynamic assessment of transurethral thermotherapy; effect versus sham procedure for treatment of BPH. Annu Meeting N E Sect AUA, Puerto Rico, 1993: 62 (abstr 16)
7. Blute M L, Tomera K M, Hellerstein D K et al. Transurethral microwave thermotherapy for management of benign prostatic hyperplasia: results of the United States Prostatron cooperative study. J Urol 1993; 150: 1591–1596

Transurethral needle ablation for treatment of benign prostatic hyperplasia

7

J. Ramon   B. Goldwasser

Introduction

Bladder outflow obstruction secondary to benign prostatic hyperplasia (BPH), with its attendant discomfort and complications, is a probability facing all ageing men. The early manifestations of BPH generally occur around the fifth decade, when it affects 50% of all subjects. From this age on the incidence of BPH increases, such that if all men were to reach the age of 90, they would all present with symptoms of BPH.[1,2]

Currently, the mainstay of BPH treatment is transurethral resection of the obstructing prostatic tissue (TURP). However, associated morbidity and mortality and the significant economic impact on the health care system have led to a search for alternative treatments.[3] Current developments and anticipated changes in the management of BPH include the following: the establishment of an improved scoring system and response criteria; transurethral implants (spiral, wall stent, intra-urethral catheter); balloon dilatation; transurethral incision; laser therapy; ultrasound-induced aspiration of tissue; heat treatment (hyperthermia, thermotherapy) and pharmacological therapies.[4]

As with TURP, these newer techniques each have their own inherent benefits and disadvantages. Such disadvantages include a lack of efficacy in a large percentage of patients, the need for a repeat or a more invasive procedure, the length of time of treatment and recovery, the high cost and unacceptable complications.[5]

Recently, a new, less invasive surgical method for treatment of BPH, transurethral needle ablation (TUNA), has been investigated.[6] The TUNA technique uses low-level radiofrequency (RF) energy to ablate tissue through the application of heat. The tissue heats up as it resists the flow of a RF current in a concentrated area surrounding a needle antenna.

In a previous study the authors assessed the feasibility and safety of the TUNA procedure in canine prostates,[6] and demonstrated that TUNA, using low-level RF, creates ablative lesions in dog prostates, which are similar in size to those reported using other methodologies without risking surrounding tissues. Subsequently, the authors investigated the effect of the TUNA procedure on human prostates. Experiments were performed ex vivo on eight prostatic adenomas that were removed during a scheduled prostatectomy. Acute exeriments in vivo were performed on five patients, immediately prior to suprapubic prostatectomy, and included the use of a built-in endoscope and transrectal ultrasound (TRUS) to control needle location. Clinical trials in vivo are now in progress. The results of all the above-mentioned studies are presented in this chapter.

Experimental results in human prostate ex vivo

Objectives

Hyperplastic canine prostate, although not an exact homologue of human BPH, is an acceptable experimental model.[7] However, before progressing to human studies in vivo, it was considered necessary to demonstrate whether TUNA treatment would elicit similar tissue responses in human prostatic adenomas. To investigate whether lesions could actually be created and to determine the TUNA settings that are appropriate for human tissues, an experiment was conducted using the TUNA procedure on prostates ex vivo.

Materials and methods

Eight patients with BPH underwent scheduled suprapubic transvesical adenomectomies. Adenomas were removed en bloc leaving an intact prostatic urethra. The specimens were treated with the TUNA device using a model ex vivo. The TUNA device included a catheter and a RF unit. The TUNA catheter was 24.1 cm long and 19 Fr in diameter with a 28 Fr bullet at the tip. The bullet contained two needles, orientated 45 degrees apart, that were laterally deployed. Each needle had a retractable shield to control the ablation area selectively (Fig. 7.1). Both the needle and the shield were advanced or retracted by controls on the catheter handle. A knob located between the catheter and handle was twisted to lock the catheter in place after rotating it into position (Fig. 7.2). Thermocouples were located at the shield's tip below each needle and at the bullet head to record ablation temperatures and prostatic urethral temperature, respectively.

The RF unit (VidaMed Inc., Menlo Park, CA, USA) included an RF generator that delivers low-power RF energy at 490 Hz, RF power level control and time set control. The unit also had the following readouts: RF power level, ablation time, impedance and six thermocouple readouts (Fig. 7.3).

The model ex vivo consisted of conductive gel placed in a metal pan that had the RF indifferent electrode attached to its underside. The excised prostate was placed upon the gel at room temperature. The two needle electrodes were deployed into the tissue of the specimen through the urethra and the protective shields were adjusted. RF power was applied at a variety of power levels for various treatment times. Tissue impedance and temperatures were recorded during power applications.

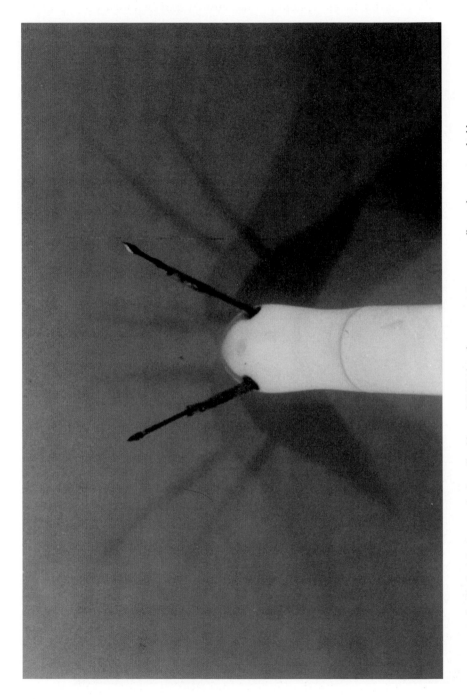

Fig. 7.1. Bullet head of the transurethral needle ablation (TUNA) catheter containing two needles and protective shields.

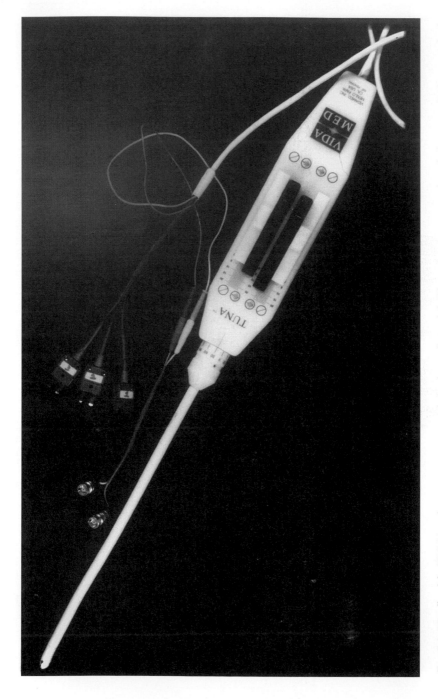

Fig. 7.2. Handle of the TUNA catheter, containing controls for the needles and shields, and connections to the radiofrequency (RF) unit. A knob located between the handle and catheter can rotate the head into the desired position.

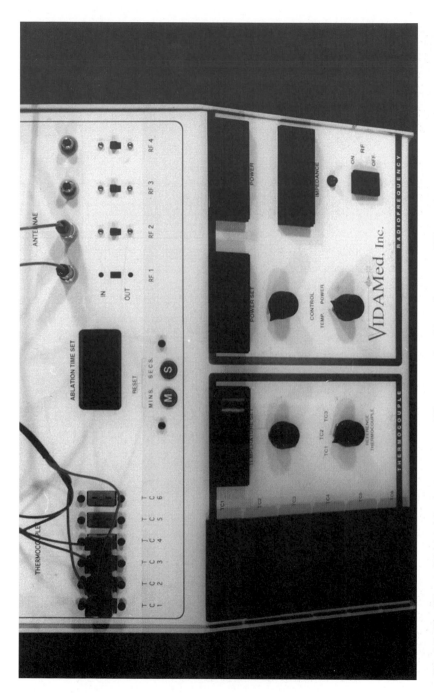

Fig. 7.3. The RF unit (VidaMed Inc.), containing an RF generator that delivers low-power RF energy at 490 Hz.

Following the experiment, the prostates were submerged in 10% formalin solution for step-sectioning and histopathology examination. The resulting thermal lesions were measured (length × width) and the morphological changes determined.

Results

Twelve applications of RF power were performed on the eight specimens using power levels of 1.5, 3, 5, 7.5 and 10 W. On average, the needle electrodes and shields were deployed at 13 and 5 mm, respectively, leaving 8 mm needle exposed (range 5–10 mm).

Specimen temperatures averaged 22°C before RF power was applied. During power application for 3 min, lesion temperatures reached 69°C on average, while the urethral temperature averaged 31°C.

As in the dogs, lesions were formed when the recorded temperatures reached 45°C and above. Such lesions were created even by very low RF outputs (1.5 W), although this took a very long time to achieve. Table 7.1 shows the average times required to reach ablative temperatures at different power levels.

RF power (W)	Average time required to reach 40°C (s)	Average time required to reach 60°C (s)
1.5	1800 (1560–2340)	2640 (2580–2700)
3.0	120 (60–180)	360 (330–400)
5.0	100 (60–170)	180 (150–210)
7.5	90 (60–150)	170 (140–200)
10.0	20 (18–24)	60 (45–70)

Table 7.1. Average times* required to reach ablative temperatures at different radiofrequency (RF) levels

*Ranges in parentheses.

Lesion temperature change increased with increasing power, while the urethral temperature change averaged 9°C (range 8–11°C). Lesion dimensions increased with increasing power at both the right and left needle electrodes, with 7.5–10 W being optimum. Lesion length correlated with the length of needle electrode exposed (6–9 and 5–10 mm, respectively). Table 7.2 shows the average effects of the RF power level on lesions and urethral temperature and the resulting lesion dimensions.

Gross examination of the prostates following RF power delivery revealed discrete lesions of greyish discoloration and tissue damage. These lesions were slender and conical in shape and rounded at the tip (Fig. 7.4). The lesions had core areas of marked tissue disruption (corresponding to the needle position) and sharp delineation from apparently normal prostatic tissue (Figs 7.5 and 7.6).

RF power (W)	Lesion temperature increase (°C)	Urethral temperature increase (°C)	Right needle lesion (mm)	Left needle lesion (mm)
3	41	11	7 × 4	6 × 6
5	43	11	7 × 5	8 × 5
7.5	46	6	8 × 5	8 × 6
10	58	8	8 × 6	8 × 6

Table 7.2. Average effect of RF power level on lesion and urethral temperature and the resulting lesion dimensions

Human prostate in vivo: acute experiments

Objectives

This investigation was mainly designed as a feasibility, safety and tolerance study. The following were investigated:

1. TUNA catheter insertion and rotation.
2. Deployment and retraction of needles and shields.
3. The ability to control the needle position within the prostatic tissue.
4. The acute effect of RF power application on prostatic adenomas in vivo.
5. Safety of treatment (complication type and rate).

Patients and methods

Five patients with BPH were treated with the TUNA device immediately before scheduled transvesical suprapubic prostatectomy. The TUNA device included a RF unit and a catheter. The RF unit (VidaMed Inc.) included a RF generator, power level and time controls, impedance readout and thermocouple readouts for catheter tip (urethral), needles and rectal temperatures.

The TUNA catheter contained two needles orientated 45 degrees apart that were laterally deployed from its tip. Each needle had a retactable shield to selectively control the ablation area. Slide controls on the catheter handle allowed for advancement and retraction of the needles and shields. The catheter also included a direct viewing fibre-optic unit which allowed precise visual positioning of the catheter (Fig. 7.7).

The procedure was performed while the patients were under general or regional anaesthesia. The patients were prepared and draped in the lithotomy position. Prostate size was measured by digital rectal examination (DRE) and transrectal ultrasound (TRUS). The TUNA catheter was advanced into the prostatic urethra and positioned using TRUS and fibre-

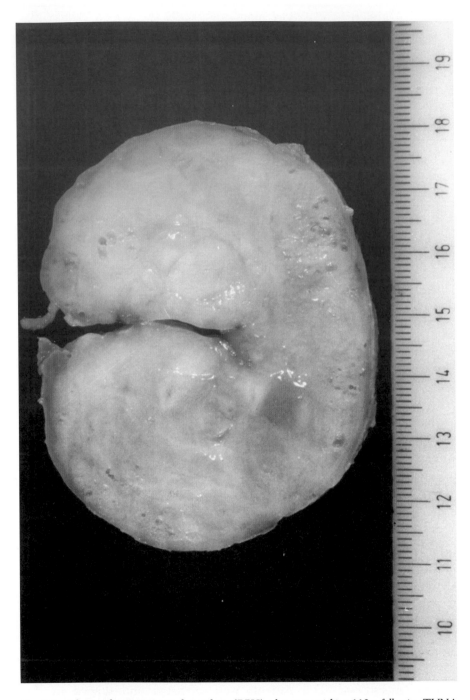

Fig. 7.4. A human benign prostatic hyperplasia (BPH) adenoma weighing 110 g following TUNA treatment in the left lobe (7.5 W for 3 min). Two ablative lesions are seen, corresponding to the position of the needle electrodes.

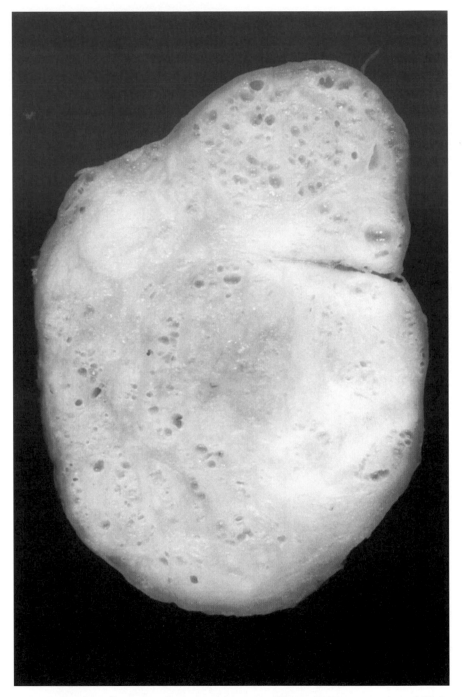

Fig. 7.5. One lobe of prostatic adenoma weighing 42 g following TUNA treatment at 5 W for 3 min. A core area of marked tissue disruption, corresponding to the needle position, is seen in the middle of the thermal lesion.

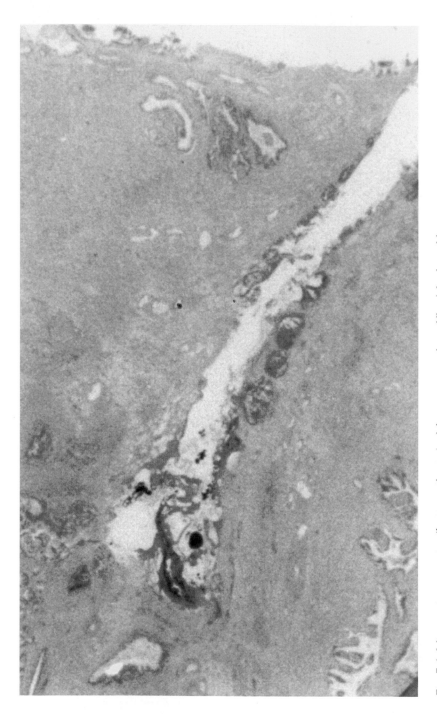

Fig. 7.6. Microscopic presentation (low magnification) of the core area in the middle of the thermal lesion.

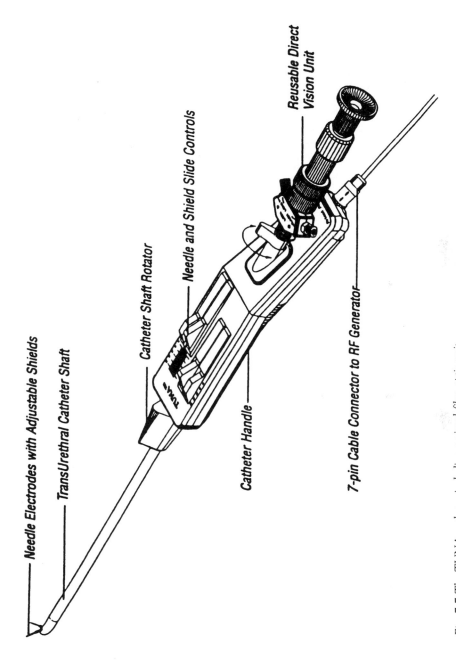

Needle Electrodes with Adjustable Shields

TransUrethral Catheter Shaft

Catheter Shaft Rotator

Needle and Shield Slide Controls

Reusable Direct Vision Unit

Catheter Handle

7-pin Cable Connector to RF Generator

Fig. 7.7 The TUNA catheter including a visual fibre-optic unit.

optics midway between the verumontanum and the bladder neck. Needle deployment was performed on both lateral lobes in that single plane.

The needles were advanced to a distance of 6 mm from the capsule and the shields were advanced to protect the urethra, leaving an average length of 10 mm of exposed needle (range 8–12 mm).

RF power of 7.5 W was applied for 3 min per plane. Tissue impedance, rectal temperature, urethral temperature and tissue temperature (measured proximal to the needle tips by thermocouples in the needle's protective shields) were recorded during RF power application. Following the procedure, the TUNA catheter was removed and the patient underwent a suprapubic prostatectomy. The adenomas were removed en bloc and were submerged in 10% formalin solution for step-sectioning and histopathological examination.

Results

TUNA catheter handling, and needle and shield deployment and retraction, were easy in all cases. Catheter position and needle position within the prostatic adenoma could be controlled using the fibre-optic and TRUS systems (Fig. 7.8).

Rectal temperatures were not affected during RF power application and urethral temperatures did not exceed 42°C. Lesions corresponding to the needle position were created. The lesions were confined to the specimens and did not reach the surgical margins. The lesions contained a core area of tissue disruption surrounded by cellular degeneration affecting mainly the cytoplasm of the cells. The cellular changes were noted within a distance of 3 mm from the core area of each lesion.

There were no difficulties in performing the scheduled prostatectomy immediately following the TUNA procedure. There were no early or late adverse effects.

Human prostate in vivo: preliminary results of clinical trials

Objectives

The objective of this phase of investigation was to evaluate the efficacy of TUNA treatment for BPH.

Patients and methods

A total of 17 men with symptomatic BPH, who were candidates for TURP or enucleation, were treated with the TUNA device, which was the same as that used in the acute experiments in vivo.

Inclusion criteria were prostate size between 15 and 75 g, International Prostate Symptom Score (IPSS) of 13 or over, peak urine flow rate less

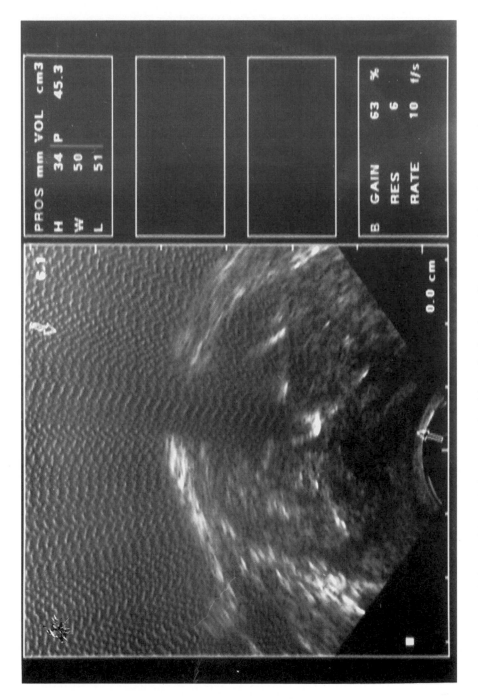

Fig. 7.8. Transrectal ultrasound (TRUS) demonstrates the ability to localize the needles accurately within the prostatic adenoma.

than 12 ml/s, and anaesthesia risk group American Society of Anesthesiology (ASA) class 1–3.

Exclusion criteria were previous prostate treatment, moderate to large median lobe BPH, prostate size greater than 75 g, confirmed or suspected malignancy of the prostate or bladder, history of bladder neck contracture and urethral stricture, blood coagulation disturbances and anaesthesia risk group ASA class 4–5.

To achieve a maximal effect by the TUNA treatment, the number of planes to be treated for each prostate was determined by the length of the prostatic urethra from the bladder neck to the verumontanum, as follows: if the length from the bladder neck to the verumontanum was less than 3 cm, the mid-plane only was treated; if the length was 3–4 cm, two planes were treated, the first 1 cm distal to the bladder neck (proximal plane), and the second 1 cm proximal to the verumontanum (distal plane); if the length was more than 4 cm, three planes were treated, namely the proximal, mid-point and distal planes.

Needles were deployed on both lateral lobes to a distance of 6 mm from the prostatic capsule. The shield length was 5 mm for a needle length of 17 mm or less, and 6 mm for a needle length between 18 and 22 mm.

Initial RF power was 5 W, increasing until tissue temperatures of 50–60°C were attained, up to a maximum of 11 W. Each plane was treated for 5 min.

The TUNA procedures were performed while the patients were sedated (i.v. midazolam). Urethral anaesthetic lidocaine hydrochloride gel was introduced into the urethra before each treatment was started.

Catheter position and needle location were monitored by the fibre-optic unit and with TRUS.

Follow-up assessment at 1, 3 and 6 months after treatment included symptom score questionnaire, sexual function questionnaire, uroflowmetry, measurement of prostate size by DRE and TRUS, urethrocystoscopy, post-voiding residual volume measurement and assessment of any adverse event.

Results

All patients were treated under i.v. sedation only. Tolerance was excellent in all cases. Average treatment time was 25 min (range 18–50 min), and was influenced by the number of planes treated per prostate.

A total of 15 patients experienced dysuria lasting from 24 to 72 h. Slight haematuria occurred in ten patients, lasting from a few hours to 7 days following treatment (average 48 h). Acute urinary retention requiring an indwelling catheter occurred in 11 patients (65%). The catheter was removed after 24 h in seven patients, after 48 h in two patients, after 72 h in one patient and after 6 days in another patient.

Patient follow-up ranged between 1 and 7 months; 14 patients were followed for 3 months. Of these, 86% (12 patients) improved in symptom score, quality of life and urine flow. Good and excellent improvement was noted in over 60% of patients. (Table 7.3). At 3 months the symptom score had improved from a mean value of 19.6 to 9.2, the mean quality of life had improved from 4.1 to 2.2, the mean peak urine flow rate had improved from 8.5 to 13.2 ml/s, and the mean residual volume had decreased from 130 to 70 ml. Improvement persisted in the four patients who were followed for 6 months. There were no late complications. All patients remained potent and none suffered a retrograde ejaculation.

Parameter	Mean change	Response at 3 months (percentage of patients)		
		Excellent	Good	Fair
Symptom score	19.6 to 9.2 (IPSS/35)	7	57	21
Quality of life	4.1 to 2.2 (IPSS/0–6)	21	29	36
Peak urine flow rate	8.5 to 13.2 (ml/s)	14	57	7

Table 7.3. Clinical trials: early results

Discussion

The experimental studies with human prostates ex vivo, treated with the TUNA device using low-level very short RF power delivery, confirmed that lesions were created, typically prolate ellipsoids formed by simple cylindrical electrodes.[8]

RF lesion generation refers to the passage of current from an electrode placed in the tissue through the surrounding tissue, thereby heating and destroying the tissue to some extent around the electrode. This method of forming interstitial lesions has been previously used in neurosurgery[8] and cardiology.[9,10] The studies described here demonstrate the feasibility of this technique in the treatment of human BPH.

Temperature is the fundamental cause of the lesion. Temperature distribution is determined by the radius of the electrode and by the increase in temperature next to the electrode's surface. The length of the tip of the electrode determines the length of the lesion. Other parameters such as lesion current, power, voltage and build-up time also affect lesion size. The RF current and power required to achieve a given temperature may vary, depending on tissue impedance, vascularity and thermal conductivity.[8]

This study demonstrated that, in prostatic tissue, ablative lesions require high temperatures, assuming 45–50°C to mark the beginning of permanent cell death. When temperatures remained below this point during RF power application, no thermal lesion was found macroscopically. Thermal lesions were always demonstrated when tissue temperatures exceeded 45°C, even if very low RF outputs were used (1.5–3 W).

The acute studies in vivo have demonstrated that TUNA is less invasive than TURP, transurethral incision of the prostate (TUIP), laser ablation or transurethral microwave ablation, because very controlled localized selective ablation of hyperplastic tissue is possible and the prostatic urethra may be left intact by raising the needle antenna shield. This ability, and the fact that no alterations in rectal or prostatic capsule temperatures occur during ablation, demonstrate the safety of the TUNA technique. Transurethral microwave hyperthermia with a cooling system produces a rise in rectal temperature (42.5°C), owing to the inability to confine microwave energy (40 W) to the desired area of the prostate.[11] The low temperature rise in the urethra (bullet temperature) using TUNA suggests that this technique may find a use as an office procedure in the future, as pain was demonstrated to be caused by an increase in urethral temperature over 45°C.[12,13]

The clinical trials have confirmed the safety and efficacy of the TUNA technique. TUNA has been demonstrated to be effective in producing symptomatic relief and increasing peak urinary flow rate. However, these results are too early to assess the long-term effects and to ascertain whether the improvement obtained by the majority of the patients will persist. Longer follow-up and further studies comparing TUNA and surgery are planned to establish the role of TUNA in the management of BPH.

References

1. Berry S J, Coffey D S, Walsh P C, Ewing L L. The development of human prostatic hyperplasia with age. J Urol 1984; 132: 474–479
2. Isaacs J T, Coffey D S. Etiology and disease process of benign prostatic hyperplasia. Prostate 1989; 12(suppl): 33–50
3. McLoughlin J, Williams G. Alternatives to prostatectomy. Br J Urol 1990; 65: 313–316
4. Khoury S. Future directions in the management of benign prostatic hyperplasia. Br J Urol 1992; 70(suppl): 27–32
5. Sarazen A A Jr, Creagh T A, Fitzpatrick J M. Alternative management strategies for BPH. In: Fitzpatrick J M (ed) Non-surgical treatment of BPH. Edinburgh: Churchill Livingstone, 1992: 3–16
6. Goldwasser B, Ramon J, Engleberg S et al. Transurethral needle ablation of the prostate using low-level radiofrequency energy: an animal experimental study. Eur Urol 1993; 24: 400–405
7. McNeal J. Pathology of benign prostatic hyperplasia: insight into etiology. Urol Clin North Am 1990; 17: 477–487
8. Cosman E R, Nashold B S, Ovelman-Levitt J. Theoretical aspects of radiofrequency lesions in the dorsal root entry zone. Neurosurgery 1984; 15: 945–950
9. Cohen T J, Chien W W, Lurie K G et al. Radiofrequency catheter ablation for treatment of bundle branch reentrant ventricular tachycardia: results and long-term follow-up. J Am Coll Cardiol 1991; 18: 1767–1773
10. Calkins H, Langberg J, Sousa J et al. Radiofrequency catheter ablation of accessory

atrioventricular connections in 250 patients: abbreviated approach to Wolff–Parkinson–White syndrome. Circulation 1992; 85: 1337–1346

11. Ersev D, Ilken Y, Simsek F et al. Preliminary results of transurethral microwave thermotherapy in the treatment of benign prostatic hyperplasia in Turkey. Eur Urol 1991; 21: 187–191

12. Astrahan M A, Sapozink M D, Cohen D et al. Microwave application for transurethral hyperthermia of benign prostatic hyperplasia. Int J Hyperthermia 1989; 5: 283–287

13. Harada T, Etori K, Kumazaki T et al. Microwave surgical treatment of diseases of prostate. Urology 1985; 26: 572–576

8

Transurethral needle ablation of the prostate (TUNA™): a new treatment of benign prostatic hyperplasia using interstitial radiofrequency energy

C. C. Schulman   A. R. Zlotta

Introduction

It is commonly estimated that nearly two out of every ten males will sooner or later require an operation to relieve symptoms due to benign prostatic hyperplasia (BPH).[1] Although surgical treatment is effective, recent data have indicated that at least 15–20% of patients undergoing a transurethral resection of the prostate (TURP) will develop a significant complication, such as incontinence, impotence, urethral stricture, or bleeding necessitating transfusion.[2] With TURP, a second intervention is necessary in 10–15% of cases within 10 years.[3] For these reasons, interest has increased in the development of minimally invasive alternative non-surgical approaches to BPH, especially in those patients who are not clear candidates for surgery or are reluctant to undergo an operation. These approaches have been encouraged by the current trend towards minimally invasive therapies, due to socioeconomic concern and patient demand. These alternatives include medical therapy (5-alpha-reductase inhibitors or alpha-adrenergic agents), or non-medical alternatives such as urethral stents, balloon dilation, laser therapy and thermal treatments. The majority of the new technologies have focused on delivering thermal energy to the prostate. Over the last few years, several studies have clinically evaluated thermal treatments.[4] Most thermal techniques involving hyperthermia (temperatures between 42 and 45°C) have shown limited efficacy and lack of objective results. Above 70°C, thermal ablation of the treated tissue is achieved. The question raised was whether an increase in the temperatures delivered to the prostate would lead to measurable lesions and an improvement in clinical results.

Transurethral needle ablation (TUNA™) uses low-level radiofrequency (RF) energy that is delivered directly into selected prostatic areas. RF heat has previously been used to ablate accessory atrioventricular bundles.[5]

Animal and human ex vivo prostate experiments

Goldwasser et al created 1 cm necrotic lesions in the dog prostate using the TUNA system with no resultant damage to the rectum, bladder base or distal prostatic urethra.[6] Similar lesions were observed in a study of the human prostate ex vivo by the same group.[7]

Transurethral needle ablation

The technique of TUNA of the prostate was explored as a rapid minimally invasive procedure that could be performed on an outpatient basis.[8] Low-level RF power is delivered directly into the prostate, through a special catheter fitted with adjustable needles placed in selected tissue areas.

TUNA achieves temperatures above 100°C in selected prostatic areas, as measured by infrared and interstitial measurements, and produces major necrotic lesions in 3–5 min. The TUNA system consists of a special 22 Fr urethral catheter connected to a RF generator. The catheter tip (Fig. 8.1) contains two needles deployed at an acute angle to each other and to the catheter (90 and 45 degree needle catheters are available). The needles and covering shields (used to protect the urethra if desired) are advanced and retracted by controls on the catheter handle. Thermosensors on the end of the shields, the tip of the catheter and eventually in the rectum measure prostatic and periprostatic temperatures during TUNA ablation. The TUNA catheter is advanced and positioned in the prostate using direct fibre-optic vision or (at the start of the studies described here) ultrasound control. By rotating the shaft with the deploying needles towards the selected prostatic area, both lateral lobes are treated in two or three planes, starting 1 cm from the bladder neck to 1 cm proximal to the verumontanum. Length of needles, and shield deployment, are determined by measuring the transverse section of the prostate using transrectal ultrasound (TRUS).

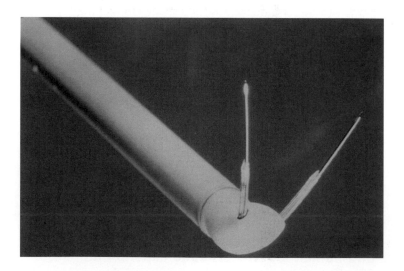

Fig. 8.1. TUNA catheter, showing deploying needles with covering shields at the tip.

Patients are treated under topical lidocaine hydrochloride anaesthesia with intravenous sedation if required. The TUNA procedure averages 30 min with a 4–15 W power applied for 3–5 min. Proximal lesion temperatures measured at the shield range from 45 to 72°C and urethral temperatures average 41°C, while central lesion temperatures are approximately 110°C, as confirmed by infrared and interstitial measurements.[9] All patients have tolerated the procedure very well. At the completion of the procedure no catheter is left in situ and patients are discharged home.

Human pathological studies

A total of 100 patients have been treated with the TUNA device in the authors' institution so far from March 1993.

An initial study on 25 patients was conducted to assess the safety, tolerance and lesions produced by TUNA. Patients were treated with TUNA before scheduled retropubic prostatectomy. Prostate weight varied from 14 to 88 g.

Macroscopic examination of the surgical prostatic specimen (Fig. 8.2) recovered from 1 day to 3 months after TUNA demonstrated localized necrotic lesions with sharp demarcation from the untreated areas.[8] These lesions averaged 12 × 7 mm and 18 × 12 mm for 3 and 5 min treatment, respectively. Microscopic examination revealed necrotic lesions with extensive coagulation up to 30 × 15 mm. Specific immunohistochemical staining showed destruction of all tissue components, glandular cells being slightly more thermoresistant than stromal tissue.

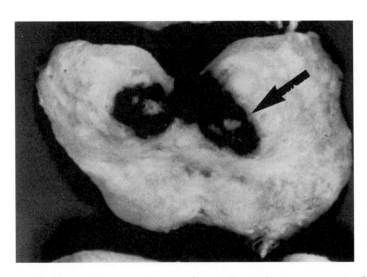

Fig. 8.2. Macroscopic appearance of necrotic lesions (arrowed) in a step-sectioned prostate specimen 15 days after TUNA.

Magnetic resonance imaging (MRI) showed necrotic lesions corresponding to those seen in the surgical specimens recovered.[10] Gadolinium contrast agent was reinforced at the periphery of the lesion and absent in the central zone of the necrotic lesion.

Clinical studies

In a clinical study, 27 patients were evaluated using the 90 degree catheter. Inclusion criteria were as follows: International Prostate Symptom Score (IPSS) and quality of life greater than 15 and 3, respectively; mean peak flow rate less than 15 ml/s (voided volume over 125 ml); post-voiding volume less than 200 ml; prostate size less than 90 ml.

Effectiveness

Symptom score and quality of life

These were assessed at 1 month, 3 months and 6 months after treatment. Table 8.1 summarizes the patient data. A significant drop was noted in the IPSS value from 20.6 (SEM 1.0) before treatment to 10.0 (SEM 1.1) at the 3 month follow-up (n=21) and 6.8 (SEM 1.2) at the 6 month follow-up (n=15).

	Follow-up period (months)			
Parameter	0 (baseline) (n=27)	1 (n=23)	3 (n=21)	6 (n=15)
IPSS value	20.6 (1.1)	11.2 (1.2)	10.0 (1.1)	6.8 (1.2)
Quality of life	4.4 (0.2)	3.4 (0.3)	2.3 (0.3)	1.5 (0.3)
Peak urine flow (ml/s)	9.8 (1.5)	13.6 (1.7)	15.1 (1.8)	15.5 (1.9)

Table 8.1. *Improvement in IPSS and quality of life amd change in maximum flow rate after TUNA*

Values are means±SEM (standard error of the mean, in parentheses).

Uroflowmetry

The mean peak urine flow increased significantly from 9.8 ml/s (SEM 1.5) before treatment to 15.1 ml/s (SEM 1.8) at 3 months follow-up (n=21) and up to 15.5 ml/s (SEM 1.9) at 6 months follow-up (n=15). Mean residual volume decreased from 71 ml before TUNA to 33 ml at 3 months after TUNA. Overall, an objective improvement in urine flow representing a 50% increase from baseline was observed in 37% of patients and a 25–50% increase was noted in 66% of the patients treated. In 30% of cases, no improvement in urine flow was observed at 6 months follow-up. In most cases, where no objective improvement was observed, prostate size was over 50 g.

Ultrasonography

Ultrasonography was performed at 30 and 90 days after treatment. Mean prostatic volume decreased from 39.6 to 33.0 g but this difference was not statistically significant. Examination of the prostate revealed, in some patients, a modification of the echogenicity (hypoechoic areas or creation of a cystic cavity) in the transitional zone, but this finding was not constant and not correlated with clinical outcome. In some patients, a TURP-like defect was seen in the areas surrounding the urethra.

Adverse reactions/complications

The most frequent complication was haematuria which occurred in all patients. Mild dysuria was noted in all patients treated, lasting 24–96 h; this was treated with anti-inflammatory agents. In 28% of patients, urinary retention occurred, lasting from 2 to 21 days (median 4 days), but spontaneously resolving in all cases. An average of 3 days was observed in 30% of these cases. No urethral stricture, urinary incontinence, retrograde ejaculation, impotence or infection was observed in this clinical series. No complaints or adverse reactions were reported at 30 days. All complaints appeared to be transient and limited.

TUNA treatment for patients in chronic retention

Twenty-eight patients in chronic retention have been treated. Chronic retention was defined as a retention due to BPH that was present for more than 2 weeks. Patients with acute retention, past history of prostate surgery, proven prostate cancer, or neurological disease, were excluded from this group. Prostate size ranged from 20 to 90 g (mean 45.5 g). Of these 28 patients, 22 (79%) treated with the TUNA procedure recovered voiding within 2–27 days (mean 8.7 days). Follow-up 6 months after TUNA (17 patients) showed a sustained mean peak flow rate at 12.2 ml/s with a mean residual volume of 90 ml.

Five of the patients who did not recover voiding after TUNA underwent surgery. Prostate size in these five patients ranged from 46 to 90 g (mean 65.7 g). Of the 28 patients in chronic retention prior to TUNA treatment, 22 voided after the procedure and clinical evaluation showed sustained improvement in urine flow at 6 months follow-up.

Conclusions

The TUNA procedure involves the use of a thermoablation device that achieves temperatures above 100°C in selected areas of the prostate, producing major necrotic lesions in 3–5 min. A major feature of this method is that it is a true outpatient procedure, performed with nothing other than urethral jelly anaesthesia and (in some patients) intravenous sedation. The low-level radiofrequency energy used with the TUNA device produces very localized, selective and controlled coagulative lesions. The extent of the lesions after TUNA exceeds all others described in reports of thermo-therapy. With the TUNA method, the size of the lesions is adapted to the size of the prostate and coagulative lesions larger than 2 cm can be created.

TUNA treatment is easy to administer and has been proved safe for treatment of BPH.

The clinical outcome after TUNA seems very encouraging, as demon-strated by the 61% mean increase in maximum flow rate at 90 days, which is a significant improvement from baseline values and findings at 30 days. The IPSS score substantially improved from pretreatment values at 3 months follow-up, and sustained its improvement at 6 months follow-up; however, a longer follow-up period is necessary.

TUNA seems to be highly effective and of particular interest in the treatment of poor-risk patients in chronic retention due to BPH and with a prostate size less than 50 g.

Apart from the high-risk group of patients who certainly can benefit from this new outpatient anaesthesia-free procedure, an increasing number of patients without absolute indications for surgery seek relief from their prostatic symptoms with minimal discomfort and complications. The low retention rate and few side effects, together with the significant improve-ment in both objective and subjective parameters observed after TUNA, make it an attractive alternative for treatment of BPH.

As with all thermal ablation devices, necrosis of prostatic hyperplastic tissue is the primary objective of the treatment. It remains unclear which part of the prostate is best sloughed for the best therapeutic effect. TUNA treatment with 90 degree needles produces lesions inside the prostate with no communication with the urethra. Pathological studies performed in the authors' institution have shown that the necrotic lesions are only 2–3 mm from the urethra, the shielding simply preventing the sloughing of the urethral mucosa and severe postoperative dysuria. The coagulative necrosis gradually changes to a retractile fibrous scar. This could result in a decrease in the volume of the treated area (although the entire prostatic volume would not change) and/or a decrease in the tonus of the periurethral tissues, hence affecting both dynamic and static components of obstruction.

Interestingly, all previous discussion regarding thermal tolerance when treating the prostate are probably outdated. Temperatures as high as 100°C have been obtained without any discomfort for the patient, even with no anaesthesia. There are probably two reasons for this absence of pain: first, there are relatively few sensory nerve endings in the prostatic parenchyma; secondly, the speed with which the temperatures are reached causes a rapid destruction of those endings.

Thus, so far, early experience with TUNA has demonstrated that this technique is a promising, easy, safe, low-morbidity, anaesthesia-free outpatient treatment for symptomatic BPH and that it produces a major improvement of both objective and subjective BPH parameters. Longer follow-up, and further randomized studies comparing TUNA and TURP, are planned to establish TUNA in the urologist's armamentarium for the non-surgical management of BPH.

References

1. Arrighi H M, Guess H A, Metter E J et al. Symptoms and signs of prostatism as risk factors for prostatectomy. Prostate 1990; 16: 253–261
2. Mebust W K, Holtgrave H L , Cockett A T K. Transurethral prostatectomy: immediate and postoperative complications. A cooperative study of 13 participating institutions evaluating 3855 patients. J Urol 1989; 141: 243–247
3. Roos N P, Wennberg I C, Malenka D J et al. Mortality and reoperation after transurethral resection of the prostate for benign prostatic hyperplasia. N Engl J Med 1989; 320: 1120–1124
4. Schulman C C, Vanden Bossche M. Hyperthermia and thermotherapy of benign prostatic hyperplasia: a critical review. Eur Urol 1993; 23(suppl 1): 53–59
5. Calkins H, Langberg J, Sousa J et al. Radiofrequency catheter ablation of assessory atrioventricular connections in 250 patients. Circulation 1992; 85: 1337–1346
6. Goldwasser B, Ramon J, Engelberg S et al. Transurethral needle ablation of the prostate using low-level radiofrequency energy: an animal experimental study. Eur Urol 1993; 24: 400–405
7. Ramon J, Goldwasser B, Shenfeld O et al. Needle ablation using radio-frequency current as a treatment for benign prostatic hyperplasia: experimental results in ex vivo human prostate. Eur Urol 1993; 24: 406–410
8. Schulman C C, Zlotta A R, Rasor S R et al. Transurethral needle ablation (TUNA): safety, feasibility and tolerance of a new office procedure for treatment of benign prostatic hyperplasia. Eur Urol 1993; 24: 415–423
9. Rasor J S, Zlotta A R, Edwards S D, Schulman C C. Transurethral needle ablation: gradient mapping and comparison of lesion size in a tissue model and in patients with benign prostatic hyperplasia. Eur Urol 1993; 24: 411–414
10. Schulman C C, Zlotta A R. Transurethral needle ablation of the prostate: pathological, radiological and clinical study of a new office procedure for treatment of benign prostatic hyperplasia using low-level radiofrequency energy. Sem Urol 1994; 3: 205–210

Heat therapy by microwaves and radiofrequency waves

9

A. Le Duc

Introduction

The predominant field of application of heat therapy by microwaves and radiofrequency (RF) waves is prostatic disease. However, some clinicians have attempted to destroy superficial bladder tumours by combined intravesical chemotherapy and local bladder microwave-induced hyperthermia.[1] The encouraging results of these very preliminary clinical studies require confirmation by controlled trials.

As far as the heat treatment of prostatic disease is concerned, clinicians have unanimously selected benign prostatic hyperplasia (BPH) for this type of therapy. The current situation regarding heat treatment of BPH can be divided roughly into two schools of thought: (a) the Israeli school, led by Yerushalmi[2] and Servadio,[3] in favour of a transrectal approach, using moderate heat of 43–44°C, and (b) the French school, led by Devonec,[4] in favour of the use of 'tropical' temperatures, exceeding 45°C, or even 'torrid' temperatures, exceeding 50°C, delivered via a transurethral approach.

Over the last 10 years, these two types of protocol have generated a wealth of literature (more than 200 articles or communications). Heat treatment of prostatic diseases is actually a revival of an older technique as, at the beginning of the twentieth century, Maximilian Stein in New York and Roucayrol in Paris used the properties of diathermy to heat or resect the prostate. A particularly courageous urologist, C. Santos, at about the same time, studied the sensation induced by diathermy in his own urethra, and concluded that this procedure 'was painless up to a temperature of 43°C, that an increasingly hot sensation was experienced beyond this temperature, which became very intense at 45.5°C, while no discomfort was experienced after 45 minutes of diathermy'. By 1920, the resistance of the male urethra to heat had been demonstrated.

It is not easy to review the current literature concerning heat treatment of the prostate, as the conclusions of the various papers range from enthusiasm to disappointment, even with the same protocol using identical apparatus. There are several possible explanations for this wide range of results. Some are related to methodology, while others are related to technology, but all are due to the fact that BPH is a disease in which objective, subjective and unknown factors are intermingled. The methodology only rarely corresponds to a randomized double-blind study compared with sham treatment. Patient selection and follow-up make little use of precise urodynamic studies, except in a few very recent studies. The scoring systems used to assess efficacy of treatment and to classify the results are often well devised, but are too individual to allow comparison of one with another. However, since 1990, this tendency has been reversed and new technological developments, such as intraurethral heat therapy, have been evaluated by well-designed studies, greatly facilitating their assessment and interpretation.

Hyperthermia/thermotherapy

A review of the literature, separating these techniques into two treatment protocols, is justified for several reasons. The borderline is situated at 45°C: treatments below this temperature correspond to hyperthermia (43°–45°C), characterized by an almost complete lack of alteration of the prostatic tissue, whereas treatments above this temperature correspond to heat therapy, in which destruction of the prostate is thermal dose dependent (see Chapter 2).

Prostatic hyperthermia

This can be applied transrectally or transurethrally. Transrectal heating is achieved by microwaves, whereas transurethral heating involves the use of microwaves or RF waves. This chapter does not distinguish between these two types of energy, but discusses the results of transrectal and transurethral hyperthermia separately.

Transrectal prostatic hyperthermia

This technique was initially proposed by Mendecki et al[5] for the treatment of prostatic cancers, and was subsequently modified by Yerushalmi et al[2] by the addition of cooling of the surface of the rectal mucosa, to treat BPH.

Numerous papers describing this procedure have been published, but very few comply with the rigorous criteria justified by the complexity of such evaluations. The recommendations of the New Technology Assessment Committee of the American Urological Association (AUA)[6] constitute a model that should be used as a basis for future studies.

As prostatism related to BPH is subdivided into two components, subjective and objective, the results are analysed here in terms of these two aspects.

Objective results

1. Prostate volume: it is unanimously agreed that the prostate volume remains unchanged.
2. Prostate-specific antigen (PSA) level: this remains unchanged, reflecting the limited cellular disruption. All studies agree on this point.[7]

3. Peak flow rate: as this objective parameter can be modified by simple urethral catheterization,[8] only studies versus sham treatment should be taken into account.

Three studies satisfy these criteria: (i) in the Paris public hospital study,[9] no improvement was found at 1 year in 150 patients; (ii) in that by Fabricius et al[10] there was no improvement at 3 months, in 51 patients; and (iii) the study by Zerbib et al[11] found an improvement of 2 ml/s better than the placebo effect in 36% of cases, in a series of 68 patients; however, patients receiving heat had displayed a significantly greater degree of obstruction than the other patients, reflecting heterogeneity of the two groups on inclusion.

Some protocols not based on a double-blind placebo-controlled design have demonstrated a very slight improvement of peak flow: Van Erps et al[12] followed 60 patients for 12 months and found an improvement of 1.8 ml/s in 35% of patients; Saranga et al[13] showed an improvement of 2 ml/s in 28% of 83 patients; other studies have shown an improvement of 1.4 ml/s in 15% of 118 patients,[14] of 1.2 ml/s in 30% of 30 cases,[15] of 4 ml/s in 59% of 34 patients,[16] and of 2 ml/s in 124 patients;[3] however, in one study of 23 patients, no change was noted.[17]

These results suggest that transrectal hyperthermia cannot be used to relieve the obstructive component of BPH.

Subjective results

Criticism concerning the lack of randomized double-blind placebo-controlled studies is even more justified when the assessment is based on an effect on the symptom score (usually the Madsen score).

A review of the previous studies reveals that, for protocols including heat versus sham treatment, no effect was found in the Paris public hospital study,[9] whereas Zerbib et al[11] noted an improvement significantly better than the placebo effect in 35% of patients (however, the same comment as before may be made concerning patient selection). For open protocols without placebo, Van Erps et al[12] found an improvement of 5 points in 68% of patients, Saranga et al[13] found an improvement of 1.3 points in 21% of cases, and Montorsi et al[14] using the Boyarsky score, found an improvement of 5 points; similarly, Kaplan and Olsson[15] found an improvement of 10 points in 60% of cases, Strohmaier et al[17] recorded an improvement of 2.5 points in 24% of cases, and Watson et al,[16] using the Boyarsky score, found an improvement of 6 points in 50% of cases.

There are obviously major differences in the results of these studies. Apart from methodological problems, Kaplan[15] also considers that a fundamental technical point may influence the results, namely, the position of the fibre in relation to the rectal wall, as well as the rectourethral distance. If this distance is greater than 2.5 cm, transrectal hyperthermia would appear to be contraindicated.

An overall view of the results illustrates the efficacy of this method; objective parameters are modified within the limits of the placebo effect, but subjective results are limited (significantly better than the placebo effect in one-quarter of patients).

Complications

Complications are rare. Lindner et al,[18] in a series of 435 patients, found haematuria in 1.4%, urinary tract infection in 1.6%, epididymitis in 1%, rectal discomfort in 1% and acute urinary retention in 0.4% of patients. Similar results were found in the series of 188 patients reported by Montorsi et al.[14] This method can be considered to be non-invasive and devoid of any real complications.

Transurethral prostatic hyperthermia

As there is no real justification for distinguishing between the efficacy of microwaves and that of RF waves, they are here considered together. The only randomized double-blind placebo-controlled study has been the Paris public hospital study.[9]

Objective results

1. Prostate volume: no modification, except in the study by Baert.[19]
2. PSA: no significant modification.
3. Peak flow: in the Paris public hospital study,[9] no significant modification was noted, taking the placebo effect into account; however, in other studies improvements were noted, of 3.6 ml/s in 80% of 63 patients,[20] of 3 ml/s in 33% of 74 patients,[19] and of 6 ml/s in 81% of 21 patients.[21] In studies using RF waves, improvements of 2 ml/s were noted in 45% of 50 cases,[22] and of 3 ml/s in 55% of 19 cases;[16] however, also using RF waves, Meier et al[23] found no change in 44 patients except in the subgroup of patients with a peak flow less than 10 ml/s.

These results suggest that efficacy in terms of relief of obstruction is difficult to assess, which means that it is limited and only concerns a small percentage of patients. Approximately 25% of patients obtained an effect superior to the placebo effect.

Subjective results (expressed in terms of the Madsen symptom score)

In the Paris public hospital study[9] the decrease (improvement) in Madsen score, although only moderate, was better than that observed in the placebo group, in 35% of cases. Other studies recorded improvements of 6 points in 92% of patients,[20] of 6 points in 80% of patients[21] and of 5 points in 75% of cases;[19] in the latter study, the presence of a prominent median lobe decreased the quality of the results and was considered by the authors to constitute a contraindication. In two studies involving RF waves, improvements in the Madsen score were noted, of 4 points in 45% of cases[16] and of 3 points for 70% of patients treated.[21]

Thus, transurethral hyperthermia has an identifiable action, constantly observed in all trials, resulting in a reduction of Madsen score by approximately 5 points.

Complications

Complications, all minor in nature, have included urethral pain and vesical spasms during treatment, urethral bleeding, increased risk of infection in the case of repeated treatments, and transient acute urinary retention in 7% of cases.

Comparison of transurethral and transrectal hyperthermia reveals that these two techniques have an acceptable morbidity and a low complication rate, with a slight advantage in favour of the transrectal approach. In very few patients (8%) was the condition exacerbated by treatment.[11]

The choice is more difficult in terms of efficacy, as neither technique is sufficiently effective. The transrectal approach appears to induce relief of the symptoms of prostatism, but the difference in relation to the placebo effect is minimal. It is also obvious that this technique cannot be used to alleviate obstruction (when it is present). The transurethral approach appears to reduce the symptoms in the same proportion of patients, with a slightly better performance on objective criteria. The lack of randomized double-blind placebo-controlled studies makes critical analysis very difficult.

Thermotherapy

This technique uses microwaves applied to the prostatic urethra to heat the prostatic tissue to high temperatures (45–80°C). The leading apparatus in this field is the Prostatron. A number of papers have been published concerning the use of this apparatus, including some reports of the results of multicentre, randomized placebo-controlled studies. Most of these studies were performed with software (Prostasoft 2) allowing temperatures of 45–55°C to be attained. However, some machines use RF waves to achieve temperatures of the order of 48°C.

Objective signs

1. Prostate volume: no significant reduction in prostate volume has been reported.
2. PSA: a constant rise in PSA, sometimes considerable, is observed during the weeks following treatment, reflecting cellular destruction. However the return of PSA to its initial value confirms that there is no significant reduction in prostate tissue mass.

3. Peak flow: a moderate improvement was observed consistently: this increase was of 3 ml/s in 64 patients, 38 reviewed at 12 months,[24] of 4 ml/s in 221 patients, 84 reviewed at 12 months,[25] of 2 ml/s in 129 patients, 48 reviewed at 12 months[26] and of 3 ml/s in 132 patients reviewed at 6 months.[27] Furthermore, micturition was restored in 21 of 25 patients with urinary retention treated by transurethural microwave thermotherapy (TUMT).[27] Of 824 patients participating in a multi-centre study,[28] 187 were reviewed at 12 months, and showed an improvement of 3 ml/s. In a study involving a rapid 1 h protocol, 64 patients reviewed at 4 months showed an improvement of 2 ml/s after therapy with RF waves at a temperature of 48°C.[29] Furthermore, three of four placebo-controlled studies reported an improvement of peak flow.[30–32]

These studies are interesting as they confirm that double-blind protocols can be conducted. The percentage error of the patients (i.e. their inability to distinguish between the treatments heat or placebo) is sufficiently great to validate these protocols.

Another aspect illustrated by these studies is assessment of the effect of sham treatment on the objective signs, especially peak flow which is modified by 1–2 ml/s; this effect has already been demonstrated by Lepor et al.[8] However, as a result of their study, Mulvin et al[33] reached different conclusions from the authors of the other four studies, with no difference between TUMT and placebo; however, it should be noted that this was the only non-randomized study. Overall, an objective although moderate effect is observed on peak flow, in the vicinity of +3 ml/s, to be deducted from the placebo effect (1–3 ml/s).

Subjective signs

Various studies have demonstrated persistent improvements in the Madsen score after heat therapy of 9 points[24], 7 points[25] and 6 points[26] at 12 months, and of 8 points at 6 months[27] and 12 months.[28] After a 1 h protocol (RF waves at 48°C) an improvement of 9 points was noted.[29]

Analysis of studies that include comparison with the placebo effect is perplexing, as the influence of this effect varies greatly from one series to another: thus de la Rosette et al[30] recorded a placebo effect of 5 points, Blute et al[31] recorded one of 4 points and Ogden et al[32] one of 1.5 points; using the WHO symptom score (WHOSS), Mulvin et al.[33] recorded a placebo effect of 10 points. Overall, the average reduction of the score symptom by heat therapy is twice that of the placebo effect (except in Mulvin's non-randomized study).[33]

Complications

Some complications are related to insertion of the catheter; others are attributable to heat. Patient discomfort during the treatment session may constitute a drawback. However, as a result of cooling of the urethral mucosa, this procedure does not require anaesthesia, but simply intravenous sedation. Urethral bleeding is usually observed for 2–3 days but is seldom severe enough to warrant readmission. Acute urinary retention is observed in 25% of patients and necessitates catheter drainage for about 1 week.

Progress in thermotherapy

Some clinicians have suggested that higher temperatures (50–80°C) might improve the effect on obstruction. Increasingly sophisticated instruments are now able to deliver higher temperatures. However, to protect the urethra and rectum, an automatic safety device that makes it impossible to burn any adjacent organs is necessary. Pathological and clinical studies have demonstrated that it is possible to achieve complete destruction of part of the prostate at temperatures exceeding 60°C.[4,34]

Three recent studies have provided preliminary clinical results of the application of high temperatures to the prostate. All three studies used the Prostatron with Software 2.5. In that by Carter and Ogden[35] the baseline peak flow was doubled; Perrin et al,[36] in a multicentre study comparing two series of patients treated at either 50°C or at a temperature exceeding 60°C, demonstrated marked alleviation of obstruction for the second group; and de la Rosette et al[30] obtained an improvement of peak flow, increasing from 9.5 to 15.5 ml/s. However, each study revealed the same drawback—a dramatic increase in adverse effects: there was marked patient discomfort, requiring potent analgesics, and the incidence of acute urinary retention was almost constant (close to 80%). Bioengineers and clinicians obviously need to find solutions in order to avoid, or at least to reduce the severity of, these adverse effects.

Conclusions

The set of symptoms referred to as prostatism is the result of complex interactions between prostatic tissue, bladder neck, detrusor and natural ageing of the lower urinary tract. It is virtually impossible to establish a reliable and simple correlation between the objective and subjective components of prostatism and the state of the prostate gland which, by its very nature, is heterogeneous, and there is obviously no simple therapeutic solution to prostatism. The development of new treatment modalities has drawn the attention of urologists to this complexity, leading them to discard the simplistic therapeutic plan, consisting of either endoscopic resection or nothing at all.

In the years to come, urologists must try to ensure a more rigorous selection of patients in order to distinguish between patients without obstruction, patients with moderate obstruction and those that are severely obstructed. Simple clinical examination completed by peak flow and determination of the post-voiding residual certainly allows an experienced urologist to establish this preliminary selection, but this is not sufficient, especially if a machine is available to treat the prostate by heat. Precise classification of patients is necessary in order to avoid successive attempts, in the same patient, with the various types of treatment available, from the least invasive to the most aggressive. The economic implications of such an approach are obviously not compatible with current attempts to reduce health expenditure.

The studies conducted by Hofner et al[37] and Dahlstrand et al[38] suggest that the most effective method of assessment of the degree of obstruction is evaluation of the voiding bladder pressure. Classification of patients on this basis, according to their degree of obstruction, allows a better selection of patients with BPH.

The major advantage of heat therapy for BPH is its beneficial effect on the symptom score. In contrast, the improvement in the objective score is considerably less. In order to improve this objective score, temperatures exceeding 50°C must be applied, with the corollary of an increased incidence of adverse effects, some of which, such as acute urinary retention, are particularly unpleasant. The use of higher temperatures must therefore be justified by the need to alleviate destruction. However, is it necessary to try to emulate transurethral resection (TURP), which creates a 'non-physiological' patency in elderly men? Why try to obtain a peak flow of 20–25 ml/s in men over the age of 60 years when the physiological normal value at this age is 13 ml/s? This question remains unanswered.

Heat therapy of symptoms related to BPH has become a reality that cannot be ignored. Although no ideal instrument exists at present, the one that most closely satisfies the therapeutic requirements of a urologist preferring this type of treatment must provide a temperature range extending from the limits of hyperthermia to the highest values of heat treatment. This instrument must also be equipped with all necessary safety devices, especially in the case of high-temperature treatments. To the author's knowledge, only those instruments with an intraurethral transmitter possess these characteristics.

Although heat treatment of symptoms related to BPH is now a reality, the duration of remission of symptoms remains unknown. An answer will not be available until the year 2000, which is, however, rapidly approaching.

Transurethral needle ablation and BPH

The principle of transurethral needle ablation (TUNA), which differs completely from that of all previously described techniques, deserves special mention. The technique most closely related to TUNA is the interstitial laser technique (neodymium:yttrium aluminium garnet or diode).

The equipment consists of a 22 Fr catheter, 25.4 cm long, connected to a 490 Hz RF generator. The tip of the catheter (28 Fr) contains two needles that can be deployed in different directions; this tip can also be rotated. All controls are located on a single panel. The needles are protected by a sheath; needles and sheaths can be advanced or withdrawn individually. The needle tips act like active electrodes, while a neutral electrode is applied to the patient's back. The intraprostatic, urethral and rectal temperatures are recorded.

The mechanism of action of RF waves is based on increased tissue resistance in response to changes in electrolytes; this increases the temperature of the tissue. The tissue lesions depend on the degree of heat, they are observed at temperatures above 50°C and coagulation necrosis occurs at a temperature of about 100°C.

Two teams have studied the size of the necrotic zone in the prostate in vivo and have reached different conclusions. According to Schulman et al,[39] an ideal oval zone of macroscopic necrosis is created around the needle at 100°C; this zone measures 17×10 mm with tissue modifications extending as far as 35×15 mm. However, according to Ramon et al,[40] there is a limiting factor: at 100°C there is charring of tissues, which insulates the needle and prevents spread of necrosis. For Ramon et al, a better therapeutic sequence is 5–7.5 W for 3 min.

The procedure is performed under intravenous sedation and topical anaesthesia. The operator treats a variable number of zones, depending on the morphology of the prostate. Needles are positioned in the gland under dual endoscopic and ultrasonographic guidance.

Clinical results have been reported by one team only:[39] in their series of 40 treated patients reviewed at 6 months, the peak flow increased from 9 to 15.8 ml/s and the WHOSS decreased from 23.1 to 8. However, these results are only preliminary and must be interpreted with caution. Studies conducted according to the criteria of good clinical practice are essential in order to assess the value of TUNA.

References

1. Rigatti P, Lev A, Colombo R. Combined intravesical chemotherapy with Mitomycine C and local bladder microwave-induced hyperthermia as a preoperative therapy for superficial bladder tumors. Eur Urol 1991; 20: 204–210
2. Yerushalmi A, Fishelovitz Y, Singer D et al. Localized deep microwave hyperthermia in the treatment of poor operative risk patients with benign prostatic hyperplasia. J Urol 1985; 133: 873–876
3. Servadio C, Braf Z, Siegel Y et al. Hyperthermia of the benign prostate. A 1 year follow-up. Eur Urol 1990; 18: 169–177
4. Devonec M, Ogden C, Perrin P, St-Clair Carter S. Clinical response to transurethral microwave thermotherapy is thermal dose dependant. Eur Urol 1993; 23: 267–274
5. Mendecki J, Friedenthal E, Bostein C et al. Microwave applicators for localized hyperthermia treatment of cancer of the prostate. Int J Rad Oncol Biol Phys 1980; 6: 1583–1589
6. AUA New Technology Assessment Committee. Guidance for clinical investigations of devices used for the treatment of benign prostatic hyperplasia. J Urol 1993; 150: 1588–1590

7. Lindner A, Siegel Y I, Korczak D. Serum prostate specific antigen levels during hyperthermia treatment of benign prostatic hyperplasia. J Urol 1990; 144: 1388–1390

8. Lepor H, Sypherd D, Machi G, Derus J. Randomized double blind study comparing the effectiveness of balloon dilatation of the prostate and cystoscopy for the treatment of symptomatic benign hyperplasia. J Urol 1992; 147: 639–641

9. Abbou C, Colombel M, Payan C et al. Transrectal and transurethral hyperthermia versus sham to treat benign prostatic hyperplasia: a double blind, randomized, multicentric study. Proceeding of the 89th Annual Meeting AUA, San Francisco. J Urol 1994; 151: 761A

10. Fabricius P G, Schafer J U, Schmeller N, Chaussy C. Efficacy of transrectal hyperthermia for benign prostatic hyperplasia: a placebo-controlled study. J Urol 1991; 145: 363A

11. Zerbib M, Steg A, Conquy S et al. Localized hyperthermia versus the sham procedure in obstructive benign hyperplasia of the prostate: a prospective randomized study. J Urol 1992; 147: 1048–1052

12. Van Erps P M, Dourcy B, Denis L J. Transrectal hyperthermia in benign prostatic hyperplasia. J Urol 1991; 145: 263A

13. Saranga R, Matzkin H, Braf Z. Local microwave hyperthermia in the treatment of benign prostatic hypertrophy. Br J Urol 1990; 65: 349–353

14. Montorsi F, Gallib L, Guazzoni G et al. Transrectal hyperthermia of benign prostatic hyperplasia: long term clinical, pathological and ultrastructural patterns. J Urol 1992; 148: 321–325

15. Kaplan S A, Olsson C A. Microwave therapy in the management of men with prostatic hyperplasia: current status. J Urol 1993; 150: 1597–1602

16. Watson G., Perlmutter A A, Shah T, Barnes D. Heat treatment for severe symptomatic prostatic outflow obstruction. World J Urol 1991; 9: 7–11

17. Strohmaier W, Bichler K H, Fluchter S H, Wilbert D M. Local microwave hyperthermia of benign prostatic hyperplasia. J Urol 1990; 144: 913–917

18. Lindner A, Siegel Y, Saranga R et al. Complications in hyperthermia treatment of benign prostatic hyperplasia. J Urol 1990; 144: 1390–1393

19. Baert L, Ameye F, Oyen R et al. Transurethral microwave hyperthermia for benign prostatic hyperplasia: preliminary clinical and pathological results. J Urol 1990; 144: 1383–1387

20. Petrovicht Z, Aneye F, Pike M et al. Relationship of response to transurethral hyperthermia and prostate volume in BPH patients. Urology 1992; 40: 317–321

21. Boyd S D, Spozink M D, Astrahan M A. Microwave hyperthermia for the treatment of benign prostatic hyperplasia. Probl Urol 1991; 5: 441–448

22. Schulman C C, Van den Bossche M, Noel J C. Transurethral hyperthermia for benign prostatic hypertrophy. World J Urol 1991; 9: 2–6

23. Meier A H P, Weill E H J, Van Waalw J K et al. Transurethral radiofrequency heating of thermotherapy for benign prostatic hypertrophy. A prospective trial in 65 consecutive cases. Eur Urol 1992; 22: 39–43

24. Carter S, Ogden C, Patel A, Ramsay J. Long-term transurethral microwave thermotherapy for benign prostatic obstruction. In: Guiliani L, Puppo P (eds) Urology. Bologna: Monduzzi Editore, 1992

25. Tubaro A, Paradiso Galatioto G, Trucchi A et al. Transurethral microwave thermotherapy in the treatment of symptomatic benign prostatic hyperplasia. Eur Urol 1993; 23: 285–291

26. Laduc R, Bloem F A G, Debruyne F. Transurethral microwave thermotherapy in symptomatic benign prostatic hyperplasia. Eur Urol 1993, 23: 202–208

27. Robinette M A, Mahoney J E, Buckley R J et al. Results of transurethral microwave thermotherapy (TUMT) in patients with symptomatic BPH and urinary retention. Proceeding of the 89th Annual Meeting AUA, San Francisco. J Urol 1994; 151: 754A

28. Devonec M, Tomera K, Perrin P. Transurethral microwave thermotherapy (TUMT) in benign prostatic hyperplasia. Multicenter study. In: Guiliani L, Puppo P (eds) Urology. Bologna: Monduzzi Editore, 1992: 239–245

29. Bhanot S M, Hargreave T B, Chisholm G D. Experience with trans-urethral radio frequency thermotherapy for benign prostatic hyperplasia and a randomised comparative study of slow 3 hours and rapid 1 hour treatment protocol. Proc 23rd Cong SIU, Sydney, 1994: A7

30. De la Rosette J J M, De Wildt M J, Alvizatos G et al. Transurethral microwave thermo-therapy in benign prostatic hyperplasia: placebo versus TUMT. Urology 1994; 44: 58–63

31. Blute M L, Patterson D E, Segura J W et al. Transurethral microwave thermotherapy vs sham: a prospective double-blind randomized study. Proceeding of the 89th Annual Meeting AUA, San Francisco. J Urol 1994; 151: 752A

32. Ogden C W, Reddy, Johnson H et al. Sham versus transurethral microwave thermotherapy in patients with symptoms of benign prostatic bladder outflow obstruction. Lancet 1993; 341: 14–17

33. Mulvin D, Creagh T A, Kelly D et al. Transurethral microwave thermotherapy versus transurethral catheter therapy for benign prostatic hyperplasia. Eur Urol 1994; 26: 6–9

34. Larson T R, Corick A A, Bostwick D. Extent of thermal cell death correlated to accurate interstitial temperatures of ten pathologic prostate specimens using urologic T3 microwave transurethral thermal therapy unit. Proc 11th Congr European Assoc Urology, Berlin, 1994: A638

35. Carter S, Ogden C. Intraprostatic temperature v. clinical outcome in TUMT: is the response heat-dose dependent? Proceeding of the 89th Annual Meeting AUA, San Francisco. J Urol 1994; 151: 756A

36. Perrin P, Devonec M, Houdelette P et al. Single session transurethral microwave thermotherapy: a comparison of two therapeutic modes in a multicenter study. Proc 11th Congr European Assoc Urology, Berlin, 1994: A640

37. Hofner K, Kramer G, Kuczyk M et al. The changes of outflow obstruction and bladder power utilisation after transurethral microwave thermotherapy. Proceeding of the 89th Annual Meeting AUA, San Francisco. J Urol 1994; 151: 757A

38. Dahlstrand C, Walden M, Petteson S, Shafer W. Pressure flow studies in BPH patients: a useful tool for treatment selection. Proceeding of the 89th Annual Meeting AUA, San Francisco. J Urol 1994; 151: 1123A

39. Schulman C C, Zlotta A R, Matos C et al. Transurethral needle ablation (TUNA) of the prostate: clinical and pathological study of a new office procedure for treatment of benign prostatic hyperplasia (BPH). Proceeding of the 89th Annual Meeting AUA, San Francisco. J Urol 1994; 151: 762A

40. Ramon J, Goldwasser B, Shenfeld O et al. Needle ablation using radiofrequency current as a treatment of benign prostatic hyperplasia: experimental results in ex vivo human prostate. Eur Urol 1993; 24(3): 400

Destruction of superficial bladder tumours with focused extracorporeal pyrotherapy

10

G. Vallancien   M. Harouni   B. Guillonneau
B. Veillon

Introduction

The use of the mechanical energy generated by focal ultrasound waves has been tested for many years since the discovery of the piezoelectricity phenomenon by Pierre and Jacques Curie.[1] The experimental studies by Fry et al[2] on the nervous system and other studies by Hynynen et al,[3,4] Hynynen[5] and Ter Haar et al[6] have opened the way to therapeutic applications of ultrasound.

In 1988, the French electronic engineer J. Dory, with whom the authors developed the first piezoelectric lithotriptor, was commissioned to construct an extracorporeal device with the aim of destroying tumour cells and tissue using focused elastic ultrashort waves. In 1990, the authors presented the first experimental studies of that technique, termed focused extracorporeal pyrotherapy (FEP).[7] Very brief heating to high temperatures, probably associated with a phenomenon of transient cavitation, seems to be the main cause of the coagulative necrosis that is observed at the focal area.[7,8]

Patients and methods

Instrument and technique

The instrument used, the Pyrotech (Figs 10.1 and 10.2) (EDAP Company, Croissy Beaubourg, France), has been developed from a succession of four prototypes and is composed of three elements—a bed allowing maintenance of the patient in various positions, a mobile firing head composed of multiple piezoelectric ceramics with a focal length of 320 mm, activated synchronously by 16 electronic generators at a frequency of 1 MHz, and an ultrasonic central probe.

The focal area is 10 mm high by 2 mm wide for 50% power at -6 dB, and in the studies discussed here the emission power exceeded 10 kW/cm^2. The instrument is mobile in three dimensions with a precision of 1 mm. Firing times between 0.015 and 1 s can be selected. The intervals between shots are also selected, depending on the disease to be treated, from 1 to 10 s. The localization system is composed of a central ultrasound transducer attached to the firing head; this 3.5 MHz sectorial transducer has a focal length of 14 cm, which automatically recedes during firing. The transducer can be

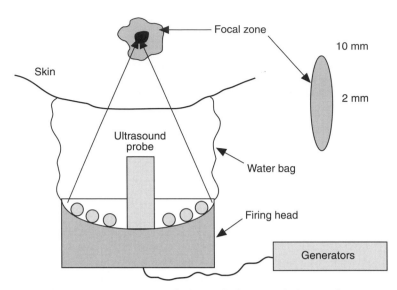

Fig. 10.1. Schematic representation of the Pyrotech device: multiple piezoelectric ceramics are placed in a semi-spherical dish and focused as 320 mm. The head is mobile. A cushion of anticavitation liquid allows the transmission of waves from the ceramics to the body. A retractable central probe allows visualization of the target.

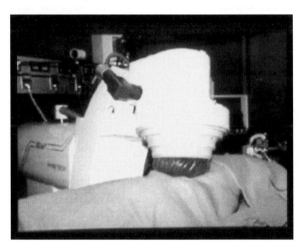

Fig. 10.2. View of the Pyrotech during treatment of a superficial bladder tumour.

orientated from the longitudinal plane to the transverse plane, passing through all of the intermediate oblique planes (Fig. 10.3). The reservoir allowing transmission of the ultrasound waves from the firing head to the human body contains a special anticavitation fluid. The control panel allows automatic displacement of the firing head[2] and mobilization by the operator, as well as selection of the shot duration and the various treatment parameters. In the event of incorrect manipulation, the security systems stop the machine immediately.

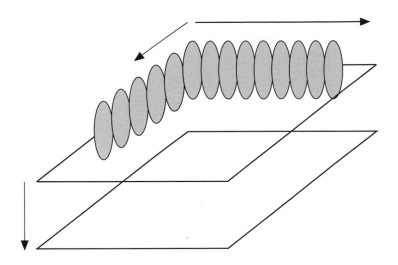

Fig. 10.3. Schematic representation of the movement of the firing head: time exposure, time interval between shots and step lengths between two shots are scheduled before the treatment. The machine starts to move longitudinally in the volume scheduled by the computer, then returns, moves laterally and starts again in a longitudinal direction. When a slice has been treated completely, the machine moves down automatically and starts to treat a second slice.

Patients

After a preliminary experimental study evaluating the liquefaction of a plastic ball placed on a pig bladder in vivo, and having subsequently demonstrated a direct effect on a human bladder tumour cell culture (line V 647),[9] it was decided to treat patients with superficial bladder tumours, for the following reasons:

1. Superficial bladder tumours are frequently detectable with abdominal ultrasound. There are often small tumours with frequent recurrences.
2. The acoustic interface between the tissues and liquid such as urine is excellent and the abdominal wall allows a relatively easy positioning of the mobile head.
3. The authors have not observed an increased risk of metastasis in an experimental study on an implanted Dunning tumour (MLL line) in rats.[10]
4. The success criteria of treatment of superficial bladder tumours are objective, combining bladder cystoscopy, bladder abdominal ultrasound, urinary cytology and eventually bladder biopsies.

Before starting this protocol, the authors evaluated the risk of pyrotherapy on 50 patients;[11] five of these patients had a recurrent superficial bladder tumour. They underwent one session of pyrotherapy immediately followed by transurethral bladder resection (TUR) of the tumour under the same anaesthesia. In all five cases a change in the appearance of the polyp was noted. In two cases, the tumour was completely destroyed and the pathological report noted a coagulative necrosis (Fig. 10.4).

(a)

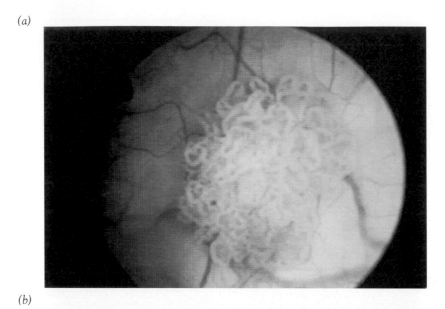

(b)

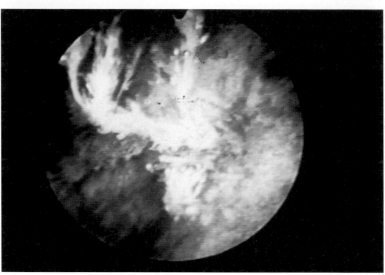

Fig. 10.4. Superficial bladder tumour of 9 mm located on the right lateral wall. (a) Pre-pyrotherapy endoscopy: the tumour is located 90 mm from the skin. A volume of 1.2 cm³ is scheduled to treat this patient. (b) Immediate post-pyrotherapy endoscopic monitoring after 210 shots on the same bladder tumour as shown in (a).

A total of 16 patients with a transitional cell tumour of the bladder were treated according to a protocol with a signed consent form. In 13 of these patients there was a recurrent tumour with a previous pathological stage PT_a–PT_1, G_1–G_2. Three patients had a primary tumour with a normal or low-grade cytology and the appearance of a superficial tumour on endoscopy.

No patient with T_3, C_{is} or infiltrated tumours were treated. General anaesthesia was required in eight patients and epidural in eight. Patients were monitored by urinary cytology, abdominal ultrasound of the bladder and fibroscopy at 1, 3, 6 and 12 months.

Results

Using the central ultrasonic probe, the authors were unable to detect the bladder tumour in two of 16 patients (12%). In one case, the tumour was on the anterior wall, with a diameter of 7 mm; in the other case the tumour was 6 mm in diameter and located on the left lateral wall in an obese patient. These two patients immediately underwent bladder transurethral resection.

In 14 patients, FEP was used without transurethral bladder resection. General anaesthesia was used in six patients and epidural in eight; the average target volume was 2.07 cm^3, the average shot duration 0.12 s, average shot number 335 and average skin target length 90 mm; average treatment time was 39 min.

Using the central ultrasonic or an endocavitary probe, the destruction of the tumour could be followed in real time, concentrating the energy beam on the bladder wall in order to coagulate the roots of the polyp. At the end of the procedure a white hyperechoic zone was noted in the bladder wall with, frequently, a shadow behind it in place of the tumour (Fig. 10.5).

Twelve patients were discharged on the morning after the procedure and two patients after 3 days. All patients had transient haematuria for an average of 3 days; one had acute retention with clots (necessitating bladder catheterization for 24 h). No patient was transfused. One patient had an abdominal subcutaneous transient haematoma (caused by anticoagulants); in the authors' opinion, anticoagulant therapy should be withdrawn on the day before FEP. One patient suffered a superficial skin burn because of a dosimetric error (failure to reduce the time exposure when the treatment head moved up to treat the superficial slice); it is planned to computerize the dosimetry.

Follow-up

Eleven patients have been followed for 1–12 months: nine are tumour free (normal urinary cytology, bladder ultrasonography and fibroscopy); two had a recurrence at 6 and 9 months. Of the original 16 patients, the remaining five were considered to be failures: these comprised the two patients without tumour visualization who immediately underwent bladder TUR, another because of a lack of power (transient breakdown of the generators) and two with only partial improvement which were considered as failures.

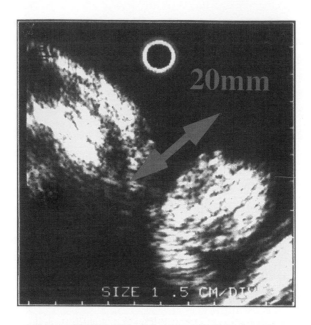

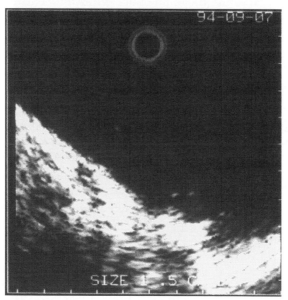

Fig. 10.5. *Endocavitary ultrasound of a bladder tumour of 20 mm diameter before (top) and after (bottom) pyrotherapy. A hyperechoic spot remains, with a shadow behind it on the bladder wall bearing witness to the effect of ultrasound on the bladder tissue.*

Conclusions

It is now known that FEP is able to destroy tumours in humans. Bladder tumour is the most objective target that can be monitored by a combination of urinary cytology before and after operation, bladder ultrasound, bladder fibroscopy and ultimately bladder wall biopsy.

The main disadvantage of this technique is the inability to provide tissue for a pathological report. Nevertheless, two facts should be emphasized: in the authors' experience of primary tumours, when cytology is normal or low grade, we have never observed a pathological report after TUR of the bladder with a stage higher than P_1; furthermore, inspection of the pathological report after bladder TUR of superficial tumours shows that in 50% of patients there is no information relating to the bladder muscle, because of the very superfical surgery. The same criticism may be made of electrocautery or laser therapy for superficial bladder tumours.

For these reasons the authors consider that, after careful selection of patients, this technique can be applied. They currently examine urinary cytology and perform a bladder cytoscopy at the consultation office before treatment. Fibroscopy enables detection of those patients with multiple small tumours, which can sometimes be undetectable with ultrasound. Ultrasound scanning of the bladder also provides much information on the most appropriate orientation of the instrument. Patients are then scheduled for hospital treatment: the procedure is carried out without further endoscopy before or immediately after operation. The first follow-up examination takes place at 1–3 months at the consultation office.

FEP has probably a role in the armamentarium of urological oncology. These preliminary results need confirmation by the experience of other teams.

Acknowledgements

The authors wish to thank the engineers and technicians of the EDAP Group, the veterinary team of the research laboratory (CERA) Fondation de l'Avenir, and Doctor Emmanuel Chartier-Kastler, Nathalie Bataille and Professor Dominique Chopin (Henri Mondor Hospital) for their help in this research.

References

1. Curie J, Curie P. Développement par pression de l'électricité pôlaire dans les cristaux hermièdres à faces inclinées. C R Acad Sci 1880; 91: 294
2. Fry F, Kossof G, Eggleton R C, Dunn F. Production of focal destructive lesions in the central nervous system with ultrasonics. J Acoust Soc Am 1970; 48: 1413–1417
3. Hynynen K, Roemer R, Anhalt D et al. A scanned focused multiple transducer ultrasonic system for localized hyperthermia treatments. Int J Hyperthermia 1987; 3: 21–35
4. Hynynen K, Shimm D, Anhalt D et al. Temperature distributions during clinical scanned, focused ultrasound hyperthermia treatments. Int J Hyperthermia 1990; 6: 891–908
5. Hynynen K. The threshold for thermally significant cavitation in dogs' thigh muscle in vivo. Ultrasound Med Biol 1991; 17: 157–169
6. Ter Haar G, Sinnett D, Rivens I. High intensity focused ultrasound—a surgical technique for the treatment of discrete liver tumors. Phys Med Biol 1989; 34: 1743–1750
7. Vallancien G, Guillonneau B, D'Avila C et al. Hyperthermie focalisée avec un système piézo-électrique extra-corporelle. Premiers Presse Med 1990; 19: 2037

8. Vallancien G, Chartier-Kastler E, Chopin D et al. Focussed extracoporeal pyrotherapy: experimental results. Eur Urol 1991; 20: 250–253

9. Chartier-Kastler E, Chopin D, Vallancien G. The effects of focused extra-corporeal pyrotherapy on a human bladder tumor cell line (647V). J Urol 1993; 149(3): 643–647

10. Vallancien G, Chartier-Kastler E, Bataille N et al. Focused extra-corporeal pyrotherapy. Eur Urol 1993; 23(suppl 1): 48–52

11. Vallancien G, Harouni M, Veillon B et al. Focused extra-corporeal pyrotherapy: feasibility study in man. J Endourol 1992; 6: 173–181

Effects of high-intensity focused ultrasound on malignant cells and tissues

11

A. Gelet   J. Y. Chapelon

Introduction

A new therapeutic option for cancer treatment, high-intensity focused ultrasound (HIFU), is undergoing clinical evaluation. Its effectiveness has been demonstrated in several types of experimental cancers implanted in rats and rabbits. Pilot studies are being carried out in humans. Preliminary results obtained from extracorporeal procedures on transitional cell carcinoma of the bladder, and by the endorectal route on adenocarcinoma of the prostate, are encouraging.

Principle of tumour destruction by high-intensity focused ultrasound

A high-intensity convergent ultrasound beam can be created either with a single focused transducer, or by a series of small transducers placed under a cupola which forms part of a sphere. The ultrasound is transmitted as bursts of ultrasound waves of a duration varying from a few milliseconds to several seconds. At the focal point of the transducer, the sudden absorption of energy by the cells situated in the target area brings about tissue destruction by a phenomemon that is not well understood.

The cellular destruction has two components. First, when the energy is of a moderate intensity for a long time (more than 1 s), a thermal effect is predominant. At the focal point a sharp increase in temperature is produced (80–85°C). This hyperthermia produces a breakdown of intracellular proteins. Conversely, when acoustic energy is delivered over a short time with a high-intensity ultrasound beam (more than 3500 W/cm^2), the tissue lesions are probably induced predominantly by cavitation.

Although both effects induce tissue destruction, it is generally agreed that, with HIFU, lesions of coagulative necrosis are caused by the thermal effect. Various research groups are therefore endeavouring to find ways of increasing the thermal effect and of reducing cavitation.

Whatever the exact nature of the destruction, the dimensions of the lesion do not exceed those of the ultrasound field when the shot is of short duration (less than 2 s). The abruptness and rapidity of the phenomenon prevents dissemination of the heat around the focal point, which explains the clearly demarcated limits between coagulated tissue and healthy tissue. As the target area is very small, it is possible to treat very precise volumes by repeating the firing and moving the transducer between each firing.

Experiments on experimental cancers in animals

Antineoplastic effect

The antineoplastic effect of focused ultrasound has been clearly demonstrated in vivo in cancerous tissues of different origins implanted in animals (Table 11.1).

It was Burov[1] in 1956 who first proposed the use of HIFU for the treatment of malignant tumours in animals and humans. Kishi and colleagues[2] reported an experiment on implantable murine glioma with significant reduced tumour growth using 1000 W/cm^2 for 2 s at 0.944 MHz.

Fry and Johnson[3] in 1978 reported an experiment on hamster medulloblastoma (implanted in rats) receiving HIFU at 1 MHz using an acoustic intensity of 900 W/cm^2 for 7 s. The tumour cure rate was 29% in rats treated with HIFU and 40% in rats treated with HIFU and carmustine.

More recently, Moore[4] and Yang[5] and their colleagues have studied the effect of HIFU on the Morris 3924-A hepatoma implanted in the ACI rat.

In Moore's experiment, HIFU was administered with a 5.5 cm diameter 4 MHz transducer, creating a continuous wave with a focal intensity of 400 W/cm^2. The tumour volume in treated animals was significantly smaller than in the control group at 4 weeks. Nevertheless, although the entire tumour was included in the target zone, no tumour was completely destroyed.

In the experiment carried out by Yang with the same tumour model, the tumour was implanted intrahepatically. The ultrasound therapy system was similar to that used by Moore. Ultrasound peak intensity was 550 W/cm^2. In an initial experiment (HIFU vs control—two groups of 56 each) significant inhibition of tumour growth was observed. On pathological examination 7–14 days after treatment, most of the neoplasm appeared to be necrotic but, in all specimens, focal areas of relatively unaffected tumour cells were observed. In a second experiment (56 ACI rats) animals were randomly divided into four treatment groups. Significantly improved survival rates were observed in HIFU-treated animals compared with control groups (control and doxorubicin alone). However, only one (7%) of the HIFU only treatment group, and 3 (21%) of the HIFU + doxorubicin treatment group achieved long-term survival without relapse or metastasis.

In 1992, Chapelon et al[6] extended the effect of HIFU to the Dunning R3327 prostatic adenocarcinoma implanted in Copenhagen rats. HIFU was

Year	Authors	Animal	Tumour	Tumour necrosis (histological study)	Reduction of tumour growth	Prolonged host survival
1975	Kishi et al[2]	Mouse	Glioma	—	Yes	Yes
1978	Fry and Johnson[3]	Hamster	Medulloblastoma	Yes	—	—
1984	Goss and Fry[10]	Rat	Sarcoma	—	Yes	—
1989	Moore et al[4]	Rat	Hepatoma	Yes	Yes	Yes
1992	Yang et al[8]	Mouse	Neuroblastoma	Yes	Yes	Yes
1992	Chapelon et al[6]	Rat	Prostate adenocarcinoma	—	Yes	Yes
1993	Sibille et al[7]	Rabbit	VX_{-2} liver tumour	Yes	—	—

Table 11.1. Effects of high-intensity focused ultrasound (HIFU) therapy on experimental cancers

generated by a 1 MHz transducer. A total of 74 rats were treated using two different sublines of Dunning tumour, and growth curves of treated animals were compared with controls. Study 1 dealt with 49 rats implanted with Mat Ly Lu subline and treated with acoustic intensities ranging from 300 to 2750 W/cm^2: complete tumour necrosis was observed in 61% of cases and only seven animals (14%) appeared to be cured without any local relapse or metastasis. In study 2, 25 rats implanted with AT2 subline were treated with an acoustic intensity of 820 W/cm^2: complete tumour necrosis was achieved in 24 (96%) of cases, and 16 (64%) appeared to be cured, whereas all rats in the control group died of progressive tumour growth within 60 days of tumour implantation.

In 1993, Sibille et al[7] analysed treatment parameters of extracorporeal HIFU in normal and VX_{-2} tumour-bearing rabbit liver. HIFU was generated with a 1 MHz transducer. In VX_{-2} rabbits, tumour destruction rates were signficantly higher in rabbits treated at 500 W/cm^2. As in the normal liver, the lesion volume increased with increasing exposure time at constant intensity.

The results suggested that HIFU therapy was capable of destroying cancerous tissues and, under certain conditions, induced a complete cure of certain experimental malignant metastatic diseases. However, it should be noted that none of the results obtained on experimental cancers are 100% perfect: in all the published series, a percentage of local relapse was observed,[6,8] or viable malignant cells were found inside the treated areas.[5] Coleman et al[9] suspect that some malignant cells can withstand higher temperatures than can normal cells. Another explanation might concern the efficacy of the shots. It is possible that the effectiveness of each shot might vary: the penetration of the ultrasound beam into the tissue could be reduced in certain circumstances, in particular by the cavitation phenomenon (the formation of bubbles at the interface between the different layers of tissue traversed). Different reasons for incomplete destruction have been described by Sibille et al.[7]

Risk of metastasis

The potential risk of metastasis induced by HIFU treatment has been studied by several authors.

Potentially, the ultrasound beam could push tumour cells through damaged blood vessels into the circulation. Fry and Johnson have observed a higher rate of secondary tumour development after ultrasound therapy:[3] in their study, tumour metastasis (which was not present in any control animal) was found in 17–44% of those treated with HIFU. This effect was not observed in all the other cases to date. In the study of Yang et al on Morris hepatoma,[5] the rate of lung metastasis was 20% in the control group and 4% in the HIFU-treated group, 28 days after tumour implantation. A similar result was observed by Goss and Fry[10] in rats with Yoshida sarcoma (metastasis in HIFU group 26% vs 43% in control group) and by Chapelon et al[6] in rats with Dunning AT2 adenocarcinoma; the metastatic rate observed in the control group (28%) was higher than the metastatic rate observed in treated rats (16%). Moreover, in animals receiving treatment, no metastasis occurred with local control of the tumour; metastatic development was observed only in animals with local relapse. It seems that HIFU therapy does not increase the risk of metastasis, but further research is needed before a definitive conclusion can be reached.

Possibly the host response against cancer may be modified after curative HIFU treatment. Dmitrieva[11] reported elimination of untreated metastatic nodules in an experiment on the Brown–Pearce rabbit tumour implanted in the testes.

Kaketa et al[12] treated rats implanted with Hories sarcoma by HIFU, and observed that cured rats developed a high resistance to subsequent tumour reinoculation. More recently, an experiment carried out by Yang et al[8] on the C1300 neuroblastoma implanted in mice, demonstrated a resistance to the development of a reinoculated identical tumour. Additional research is required to confirm whether an immune response to cancer occurs after curative local tumour treatment by HIFU.

Clinical applications in human cancer: the first three pilot studies

Three pilot studies have been completed or are in progress.

Study by Vallancien et al

The aim of Vallancien's pilot study[13] was the destruction of superficial bladder tumours with 'focused extracorporeal pyrotherapy' (HIFU delivered extracorporeally).

HIFU therapy was carried out using an extracorporeal firing head containing multiple piezoelectric elements, focused at 320 mm (Pyrotech, Edap Company, Croissy Beaubourg, France). A cushion provided the contact between the skin and the firing head. The bladder tumour was targeted and the target volume including the bladder wall was calculated. Six patients with recurrent superficial bladder transitional cell carcinoma (TCC) (PT_A G_1, PT_1 G_1 or G_2) were treated under epidural anaesthesia. The authors observed no skin burning. Follow-up at 6 months showed that four patients were free of tumours while in two cases the effect was only partial. The authors concluded that HIFU was able to destroy completely superficial bladder TCC without any endoscopic procedure and no side effects.

Study by Gelet et al

The aim of Gelet's pilot study[14] was the treatment of localized prostatic cancer by HIFU, delivered via the transrectal route.

The device to produce HIFU (Ablatherm Technomed, France) combines a 2.25 MHz therapy transducer and a transrectal biplane scanner probe (Kretz Technik, Austria) working at 7.5 MHz. A total of 14 patients (mean age 71 years) were treated using two different therapy transducers focused respectively at 35 mm (three sessions) and 45 mm (26 sessions). The clinical stage of the tumours was T_1 (three patients) and T_2 (11 patients). The mean pretreatment prostate-specific antigen (PSA) level was 12±2.6 ng/ml (Hybritech). The treatment was performed under anaesthesia, in the lateral decubitus position. In the first five patients, the volume treated was less than the overall prostatic volume; in the next eight patients the volume treated was equal to or greater than the prostatic volume. A rectal burn occurred after the first three sessions performed with the 35 mm focused transducer. Basically, the follow-up consisted of monitoring the PSA level and randomized biopsies. The mean post-treatment PSA level (Fig. 11.1) was 2.42 ng/ml (mean follow-up period 9 months). Control biopsies demonstrated coagulation necrosis lesions of the treated prostatic tissue, with subsequent development of fibrosis. No evidence of cancer was found in seven patients; residual cancer was found in seven patients, but only three required further treatment (orchiectomy in one; supplementary HIFU sessions in two).

The authors concluded that it is potentially possible to carry out

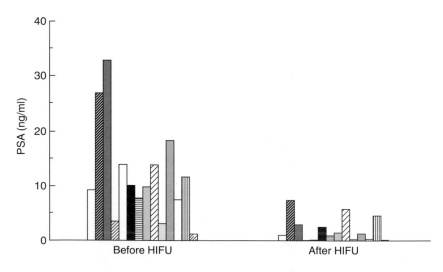

Fig. 11.1. Treatment of localized prostatic cancer in humans: prostate-specific antigen (PSA) development after HIFU treatment via the transrectal route (mean level before treatment, 12.25 ng/ml; mean level after treatment, 2.18 ng/ml).

satisfactory local control of organ-confined prostatic adenocarcinoma using transrectal HIFU in humans.

Study by Marberger et al

The aim of Marberger's pilot study[15] was the treatment of non-surgical prostatic cancer by HIFU.

The device to produce HIFU (Sonablate, Focal Surgery, USA) operated with site intensities varying from 1460 to 2000 W/cm^2. In the study, the authors, using HIFU, targeted hypoechogenic circumscribed lesions. Three patients with B_1 adenocarcinoma were treated without postoperative morbidity. Follow-up biopsies were negative in two patients (follow-up 3 months). In the third patient, residual cancer was found and further HIFU treatment was carried out without additional toxicity. The authors concluded that it seems possible to achieve local tumour destruction using a minimally invasive therapeutic option.

Discussion

Even at this very early stage, these results demonstrate that HIFU can destroy internal localized cancers. This type of treatment has several major potential advantages: (1) it is relatively non-invasive; (2) it requires only a short hospital stay; (3) it can easily be repeated, and finally (4), should the effects be incomplete, it is possible to turn to another form of treatment (radiotherapy, hormone therapy), as the neighbouring organs are not affected by the passage of the ultrasound beam.

The development of an efficient and non-invasive treatment for the numerous patients with localized cancer of the prostate would constitute a considerable step forward. The existence of a reliable gauge for the development of the cancer and the possibility of repeated control biopsies would facilitate monitoring of the efficacy of the treatment. However, in view of the multifocal nature of this type of tumour, it will certainly be necessary to treat the whole of the gland. The long-term development of the body of tissue treated is still largely unknown.

In the long term, other applications of the treatment may be put into practice (in cancer of the kidney, the breast or the liver, for example).

References

1. Burov A K. High intensity ultrasound for the treatment of malignant tumors in animals and man. Dikl Akad Nauk SSSR 1956; 106: 239–241
2. Kishi M, Mishima T, Itakura T et al. Experimental studies of effects of intense ultrasound on implantable murine glioma. In Kazner E, de Vlieger M, Muller HR, Mc Cready VR (eds) Proc 2nd Eur Congr Ultrasonics Med. Amsterdam: Excerpta Medica, 1975: 28–33
3. Fry F J, Johnson L K. Tumor irradiation with intense ultrasound. Ultrasound Med Biol 1978; 4: 377–341
4. Moore W E, Lopez R, Matthews D E et al. Evaluation of high intensity therapeutic ultrasound irradiation in the treatment of experimental hepatoma. J Pediatr Surg 1989; 24: 30–33

5. Yang R, Reilly C R, Rescorla F J et al. High intensity focused ultrasound in the treatment of experimental liver cancer. Arch Surg 1991; 126: 1002–1010
6. Chapelon J Y, Margonari J, Vernier F et al. In vivo effects of high intensity ultrasound on prostatic adenocarcinoma Dunning R3327. Cancer Res 1992; 52: 6353–6357
7. Sibille A, Prat F, Chapelon J Y et al. Characterization of extracorporeal ablation of normal and tumor-bearing liver tissue by high intensity focused ultrasound. Ultrasound Med Biol 1993; 9: 803–813
8. Yang R, Reilly C R, Rescorla F J et al. Effects of high intensity focused ultrasound in the treatment of experimental neuroblastoma. J Pediatr Surg 1992; 27: 246–251
9. Coleman D J, Silverman R H, Iwamoto T et al. Histopathologic effects of ultrasonically induced hyperthermia in intraocular malignant melanoma. Ophthalmology 1988; 95: 970–981
10. Goss S A, Fry F J. The effects of high intensity ultrasonic irradiation on tumor growth. IEEE Trans Sonics Ultrasonics 1984; 31: 491–496
11. Dmitrieva N P. Resorption of not exposed metastases following the effect of ultrasound of high intensity on Brown–Pierce tumors in rabbits. Biull Eksp Biol Med 1957; 44: 81–85
12. Kaketa K, Wagai T, Mizuno S et al. Annual report (1971). Tokyo: Medical Ultrasonics Research Center Tokyo, Juntendo University School of Medicine, 1971
13. Vallancien C, Harouni M, Veillon B et al. Destruction of superficial bladder tumors with focused extracorporeal pyrotherapy (FEP). EAU Congr Abstr 1994: 30
14. Gelet A, Chapelon J Y, Bouvier R et al. Treatment of localized prostatic cancer by transrectal route: preliminary results. EAU Congr Abstr 1994: 267
15. Marberger M, Susani M, Madersbacher S et al. Effect of high intensity focused ultrasound on human prostatic cancer. EAU Congr Abstr 1994: 266

REPORT

Therapeutic applications of ultrasound in urology

12

S. Madersbacher   M. Marberger

Introduction

Ultrasound is an acoustic mechanical wave, consisting of compressions and rarefactions, that propagates within a medium (Fig. 12.1). The ultrasound wavelength used in medicine is sufficiently short to be brought to a tight focus at depth within the body. This ability to focus means both that good resolution may be obtained in diagnostic ultrasound scans (using low-output power) and that, if sufficient energy is carried within the ultrasound beam, regions of high ultrasonic power are created in which therapeutic effects are obtained.

In general, ultrasound interacts with tissue both thermally and mechanically.[1] Mechanical interaction involves acoustic cavitation, acoustic pressure, acoustic force, acoustic torque and acoustic streaming. Thermal interaction, mediated by acoustic absorption, is the best understood and is implicated in a broad variety of ultrasonic biological effects.

Mechanical effects of ultrasound

The mechanical tissue effects of ultrasound have been recently reviewed by Barnett et al[2] in detail and some basic aspects are discussed herein.

Acoustic pressure is exerted on any body immersed in an acoustic field. In a standing wave-field, it is greatest at pressure maxima and lowest at velocity maxima. Similarly, *acoustic force* is exerted on any body immersed in an acoustic field. In a plane travelling wave-field the force is in the direction of propagation and is proportional to the intensity. Non-uniformity of the acoustic field also leads to a time-independent twisting action which is referred to as *acoustic torque*. This torque produces a rotating movement of cells and intracellular structures in the medium and may result in a spinning motion of cells in suspension or of intracellular structures. *Acoustic streaming* describes the movement of fluid in an ultrasonic pressure field. Where fluid motion encounters boundaries, high velocity gradients can develop and produce substantial shear stresses. Fluid motion around microscopic cavitation bubbles (see below) is known as acoustic microstreaming. Shear stresses at cell membranes may be responsible for changes in membrane permeability and may subsequently induce cell membrane breakage and haemolysis if a critical shear stress is

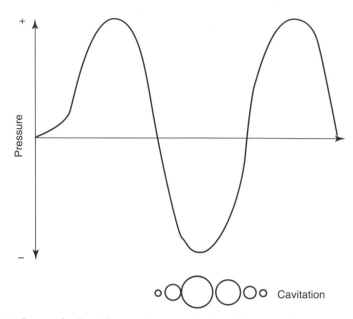

Fig. 12.1. Ultrasound pulse. Ultrasound consists of a sinusoidal wave with alternating positive and negative deflections and a well-defined wavelength. The negative-pressure portion of the ultrasound wave is considered to be responsible for cavitation bubble formation.

exceeded. The most prominent mechanical effect of therapeutic ultrasound on tissue is *acoustic cavitation*, which is defined as the formation and/or activity of gas- or vapour-filled cavities (bubbles) in a medium exposed to an ultrasound field (Fig. 12.1). Generally accepted terms for specific aspects of bubble activity are *stable* and *inertial* (collapse) *cavitation* (also known as transient cavitation). Stable cavitation describes the continuous oscillation of bubbles in response to alternating positive and negative pressure in an acoustic field. The bubble radius varies about an equilibrium value and the pulsating cavity exists for a considerable number of cycles. Inertial cavitation describes the behaviour of bubbles that oscillate about their equilibrium size, grow until the outward excursion of the surface exceeds a limiting value, and collapse violently. It is a random phenomenon and its occurrence is unpredictable, difficult to control and leads to uncontrollable tissue destruction. Histologically, cavitation is characterized by 'punched out' cavities. Acoustic cavitation is believed to be responsible for most biological effects of ultrasound on cell suspensions *in vitro*, the most likely outcome being cell death.

The mechanical effect of ultrasound is employed in contact lithotripsy, ultrasonic tissue dissection and extracorporeal shock wave lithotripsy (ESWL). The therapeutic effect of extracorporeal ultrasonic tissue tripsy ('pyrotherapy') is not fully understood, yet mechanical effects (tissue cavitation) are considered to be predominantly involved.

Therapeutic applications of mechanical effects of ultrasound

Contact lithotripsy

Contact ultrasonic lithotripsy is used to disintegrate urinary stones in endourological procedures. In principle, ultrasound energy is used to propel a steel probe to act as a jackhammer.[3] Instruments consist of an ultrasound transducer with an integrated sonotrode and an external generator. When powered at about 100 W, the piezoceramic elements in the ultrasonic transducer produce ultrasound of a frequency of 23–27 MHz (Fig. 12.2).[3] With an acoustic horn bolted to the acoustic endparts, the integrated steel probe protruding from the transducer is propelled to longitudinal and transverse vibrations, which are utilized to disintegrate the calculus on contact. Stone disruption is achieved purely by mechanical forces due to the oscillation of the probe, mainly with a longitudinal amplitude in the range of 20 μm.

The efficacy of the probe increases, the better the contact between stone and sonotrode. At disintegration the probe rapidly heats up to temperatures above 50°C unless water cooled. The system is therefore always employed under water and with a continuous-flow irrigation system. The sonotrode is usually hollow and connected to a vacuum pump to remove the irrigation fluid and stone dust simultaneously (Fig. 12.2).[3] The main advantage of ultrasonic lithotripsy lies in its minimal adverse effects on surrounding soft tissue, due to the short amplitude of the probe (20 μm). The maximum sound intensity at the tip of a sonotrode is less than 0.35 W/cm^2, and decays rapidly within millimetres from the tip, especially in oblique

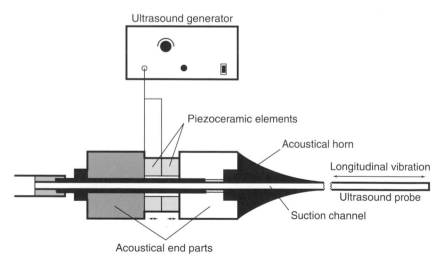

Fig. 12.2. Contact lithotripsy. Ultrasound energy is transformed into longitudinal and transverse vibrations of a hollow steel probe, which guides the energy to the focus. Good contact between the probe and stone is essential and is promoted by connecting the central lumen of the probe to a vacuum pump. (Adapted from ref. 3.)

directions, or with interposition of a calculus. As even under optimum conditions the cavitation threshold for ultrasound at this frequency is at least 0.7 W/cm^2, cavitation does not occur.

Ultrasonic tissue dissection

If the vibration of ultrasound probes exceeds 50 μm, soft tissues are disintegrated upon contact. In the mid-1960s, the first clinical studies using axial vibrations of a hollow metal needle generated by ultrasound were reported to disrupt and remove opacified human lenses. This technology is known as ultrasonic tissue dissection and operates in the frequency range of 20–50 kHz.[4-7] The resultant longitudinal motion is magnified and amplified by a connecting body and an interchangeable probe tip (Fig. 12.3); this results in a longitudinal tip excursion of 200–300 μm. The three functions of mechanical fragmentation, metered irrigation and controlled suction are incorporated in a scalpel-like handpiece (Fig. 12.3).[5,6] This vibration of the probe tip produces a purely mechanical effect by direct contact with the structure to be agitated, leading to tissue fragmentation. The cooling irrigating saline solution suspends the cell fragments, which are subsequently aspirated by the suction system. The probe heats up rapidly and requires continuous water cooling.

Soft tissues are easy to disintegrate. Ultrasonic aspiration permits dissection of soft tissue off major blood vessels and nerves without damaging these structures. This technique is in routine clinical use for

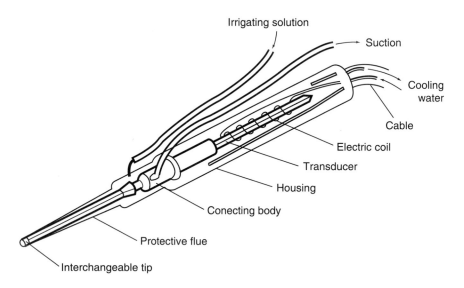

Fig. 12.3. Ultrasonic tissue dissection. The three functions of fragmentation power, metered irrigation and controlled suction are transferred from the control console through a cable to the surgical handpiece. (Adapted from ref. 5.)

extraction of cataracts as it requires only a minimal incision in the sclera. In open surgery, it has been used for the resection of brain and liver tumours;[6] it has also been applied to the removal of dental calculus.

In urology, ultrasound aspiration systems have been evaluated for nephron-sparing surgery in cases of renal malignancy,[5] but have found only limited acceptance because of the time-consuming procedure. Previous attempts to develop ultrasound aspiration systems for endoscopic procedures were unsuccessful because the long endoscopic probes were not strong enough to withstand the high amplitude. Recently, Ishibashi et al[7] reported the use of a titanium probe for endoscopic ultrasound aspiration, combined with a coagulation system. This probe has been tested in experimental settings and preliminary clinical data for endoscopic surgery of bladder tumours and benign prostatic hyperplasia (BPH) are available. Although aspiration of bladder tumours was rapidly achieved, ultrasound dissection of BPH tissue was difficult.

Extracorporeal shock wave lithotripsy

A shock wave is characterized as a single positive-pressure front that has a steep onset and a gradual decline (Fig. 12.4a). The high pressures associated with a shock wave lead to a discontinuous distortion of the leading edge of the wave.[8] In ESWL, a number of piezoceramic elements mounted on a concave disc are subjected simultaneously to an electrical discharge[9,10] (Fig. 12.4b). The resulting single ultrasound wave leaves the disc as a shock wave. As the wave travels through the medium (degassed water, tissue) its steepness increases so that it becomes a shock wave with a steep, very rapid positive increase and a very blunted negative phase, with a maximum at the focus of the system[9,10] (Fig. 12.4a). The mechanism of stone fragmentation by shock waves is not entirely understood, but two mechanisms are thought to be involved.[9] When the concave shock wave strikes the leading edge of a stone, a portion is reflected. The interface between the primary and reflected shock wave creates a strong tensile stress that literally tears off a layer of material from the leading edge of the stone. The original shock wave and the reflected shock wave create a large tensile force that also tears a layer of material from the rear surface of the stone. The passage of multiple shock waves through a stone ultimately will lead to the pulverization of the entire stone; this phenomenon is termed spalling.

If firing frequency increases to more than 10/s, significant cavitation is induced at the focal area, which leads to uncontrollable tissue damage. Consequently, the frequency of ESWL impulses is usually set below 10 Hz. Within the last decade, ESWL has revolutionized the therapy of urolithiasis and has also been applied in combination with medical therapy to treat gallstones and sialolithiasis. As this topic is not within the scope of this chapter, the interested reader is referred to the respective literature.

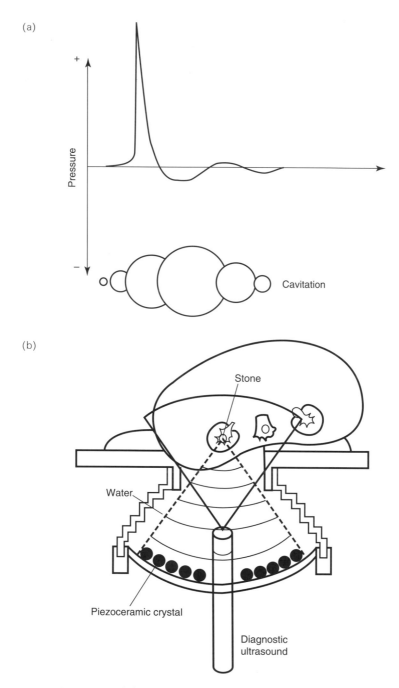

Fig. 12.4. Extracorporeal shock wave lithotripsy. (a) Shock wave pulse: this is characterized by a rapid rise and gradual fall in pressure. Cavitation bubble formation during the negative pressure phase is significantly pronounced, compared with that of the sinusoidal ultrasound wave. (b) Schematic illustration of a piezoelectric lithotriptor. Numerous small piezoelectric crystals are mounted on a spherical surface. Simultaneous activation of the crystals generates a concave shock wave that converges at the centre of the spherical surface. (Adapted from ref. 10.)

Soon after the establishment of ESWL, the impact of high-energy shock waves on benign and malignant cells was studied intensively (see Chapter 1 and refs 11 and 12). In vitro, drastic cellular alterations were demonstrable in various experimental settings.[11,12] Despite these encouraging findings in vitro, results in vivo applying various tumour models were disappointing. A transient therapeutic effect was present only if fairly slow-growing tumour models were studied; if rapidly growing tumour cells were treated, no significant therapeutic effect was demonstrable. Hence, shock wave treatment with a classic lithotriptor does not seem to induce irreversible cell damage and clinical trials have not been reported.

Extracorporeal ultrasonic tissue tripsy ('pyrotherapy')

The negative pressure of a shock can be sufficient to induce tissue cavitation within the focal zone (Figs 12.4a and 12.5a). As mentioned above, tissue cavitation can also be induced by increasing the frequency of shock wave generation beyond 10 shots/s. A combination of both mechanisms leads to massive tissue cavitation within the focal zone, sufficient to cause immediate cell death (Fig. 12.5a). Vallancien et al[13–15] recently described an extracorporeal apparatus for in-depth tissue ablation based on this mechanism (Fig. 12.5b). The system is an adaptation of a lithotriptor (Pyrotech, EDAP Company, Croissy Beaubourg, France; for a detailed description of this system see Chapter 10). The energy source comprises multiple transducer elements and has a focal length of 15 cm. The site intensity used has been quoted to exceed 10 000 W/cm^2, but precise data are not available.[13,15] A 3.5 MHz sectorial imaging transducer with a focal length of 14 cm is positioned at the centre of the therapy elements. The focal area is 10 mm high by 2 mm wide for 50% power at -6 dB. The sound head is positioned in a large bag of cavitation-free water below a waterproof membrane in the middle of a bed.[13–15]

During extracorporeal pyrotherapy, the bubble formation within the focal zone increases progressively, the bubbles subsequently collapsing rapidly. This rapid collapse leads to a compression of the gas inside the bubble without heat exchange with the surrounding tissue and results in a local temperature increase. Thus, extracorporeal ultrasonic tissue tripsy is considered to make use of both the mechanical and the thermal effects of ultrasound. However, as the predominant therapeutic effect appears to be tissue cavitation, the report on this technology was incorporated within this section on mechanical effects. This extracorporeal device has been tested under numerous experimental conditions and preliminary human trials involving prostate, kidney and bladder have been reported. Vallancien et al[13] studied sequential histological effects of extracorporeal ultrasonic tissue tripsy on 110 kidneys of white Landrace pigs. Immediately after treatment, massive congestion with haemorrhage and exsudation was present. After 24 h a coagulative necrosis appeared, on day 7 the target area

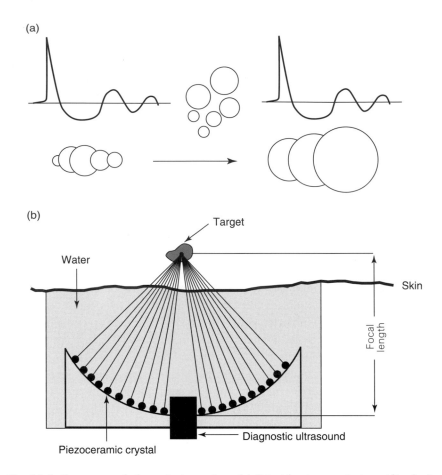

Fig. 12.5. *Extracorporeal ultrasonic tissue tripsy. (a) Principle: tissue cavitation within the focal zone can be augmented by increasing the negative portion of the shock wave and by increasing the frequency of shock wave generation beyond 10 Hz. (b) Apparatus: the firing head consists of multiple piezoelectric crystals with a focal length of 320 mm, activated synchronously by 16 electromagnetic generators. For air-free coupling of the shock wave and tissue (skin), the interface is filled with degassed water. (Adapted from ref. 13.)*

was completely necrotic and by day 90 there was fibrotic scarring of the treated area. Electron microscopy of the target area revealed the complete destruction of all intracytoplasmatic organelles, such as ribosomes, Golgi apparatus and mitochondria.

In humans, the histological impact of extracorporeal ultrasonic tissue tripsy on renal tissue has recently been investigated. Patients with renal cancer (n=5), renal atrophy (n=2) and complex stones (n=1) were subjected to extracorporeal ultrasonic tissue tripsy before nephrectomy.[14,15] The mean treated volume was 4 cm^3, the mean number of shots was 195 and the average distance between the skin and the focal point was 68 mm. Immediately after the procedure, treated areas showed intense congestion with severe hyperaemia and marked alterations of the microcapillaries. These results were identical to those observed in the pig kidney.[13] After 48 h, early signs of limited subcapsular necrosis with a persistent zone of hyperaemia were detected. Side effects were moderate: two patients noted skin burns, but no other significant adverse effects were seen. During surgery, moderate oedema of the perirenal fat was observed in two cases; no subcapsular or perirenal haematomas were present.

Extracorporeal ultrasonic tissue tripsy has also been applied to the ablation of prostatic tissue.[14,15] Although intraprostatic coagulative necrosis was demonstrable, the transabdominal approach proved to be poorly suited because the prostate is shielded by the bony pelvis. Vallancien et al[14,15] could target the prostate adequately in only 50% of cases. As Chapter 10 reports experimental and clinical data for bladder tumours, this issue is not discussed here.

Thermal effects of ultrasound

As an ultrasound wave propagates through a medium, it is progressively absorbed and the energy is converted to heat in any not ideally viscoelastic medium, such as all biological tissues. In diagnostic ultrasound systems, the amount of heat generated is extremely small and has not been shown to have any harmful effect. In therapeutic systems, high intensities are used so that significant temperature elevations are achieved that affect the tissues.[1]

The thermal effect of ultrasound on tissue is dependent on a number of factors, including the following:

1. Ultrasonic site intensity throughout the insonified tissues.
2. Absorption coefficient of the tissues insonicated.
3. The temperature rise throughout the exposed tissues: for short time intervals (less than 0.1 s) the temperature rise is proportional to the ultrasonic intensity. As time increases, temperature rises are modified by thermal conduction and the simple proportionality is no longer valid. In perfused tissues, blood-flow cooling is an important additional factor.
4. The damage index estimating the effects of temperature elevation on tissue structures: tissue changes occur if the heat induction exceeds the threshold level of protein degradation of 45–47°C.

High-intensity focused ultrasound

A beam of ultrasound may be brought to a tight focus at a selected depth within the body, thus producing a region of high energy density within which tissue can be destroyed without damage to overlying or intervening tissue. This technique is known as ultrasound ablation, focal ultrasound surgery or high-intensity focused ultrasound (HIFU): this chapter employs the latter term (for review see refs 16 and 17).

This technique was firmly established in the mid-1950s by the pioneering work of Frank and William Fry and was initially used to ablate brain tissue.[18,19] Subsequent years have seen steady progress in understanding the basic physical principles involved in the interaction of this mechanical waveform with biological tissue. In parallel, progress in transducer technology and the advent of new powerful diagnostic tools, such as high-frequency ultrasonography and magnetic resonance imaging (MRI), have been the technological basis for recent designs of devices. These developments have resulted in the initiation of human trials involving several organs.

The source of HIFU is a piezoceramic transducer, which has the property of changing its thickness in response to an applied voltage. This creates an acoustic ultrasound wave with a frequency equal to that of the voltage applied. Frequencies used for HIFU therapy cover a range of 0.5–10 MHz.[16,17] The site intensity applied has to be above the temperature threshold, yet below the cavitation threshold to avoid damage to surrounding structures and usually ranges between 750 and 4500 W/cm^2. The focusing of the HIFU beam is achieved either by placing a lens in front of the transducer, or using a concave transducer.[17] Modern piezoceramics can operate at sufficient power densities with long-term output stability to conform to focal therapy device requirements. Coupling of the transducer to the tissue of interest must exclude air and usually involves low-loss media that do not absorb ultrasound energy, such as degassed water. The shape of the focal zone can change significantly with focal length, exposure time and site intensity, as was recently demonstrated in vitro by Ter Haar et al.[20]

HIFU instrumentation

At present, two types of HIFU systems are available—transrectal or extracorporeal. The transrectal devices were designed to ablate prostatic tissue and incorporate a small imaging and therapy transducer on a single probe sheath (Fig. 12.6a,b). For air-free coupling of the HIFU beam to rectal wall tissue, the probe is covered by a condom, which is filled with degassed water after insertion into the rectum. In one device (Sonablate, Focal Surgery Inc., Milpitas, USA) the same 4.0 MHz transducer is used for imaging and therapy (Fig. 12.6a).[21–23] The focal length is dependent on the crystal used; currently, individual focal lengths of 2.5, 3.0, 3.5 and 4.0 cm are available. The site intensity can be varied from 1260 to 2200 W/cm^2. A 4 s interval of therapy (=power on), followed by 12 s power off, is used for obtaining an image update and moving the transducer electronically to the next treatment location.[21–23] The second transrectal device (Ablatherm, Technomed International, Lyon, France) uses two separate transducers, one for imaging operating at 7.5 MHz and one for HIFU therapy at 2.25 MHz (focal length 3.5 cm) (Fig. 12.6b).[24] Site intensities in this system have been reported to range between 700 and 2200 W/cm^2.

Extracorporeal HIFU devices were designed for transcutaneous in-depth tissue ablation of organs accessible to ultrasound. The first extensive human applications of HIFU were in the mid-1950s, for ablation of brain tissue. The HIFU transducer consisted of four firing heads, each provided

(a)

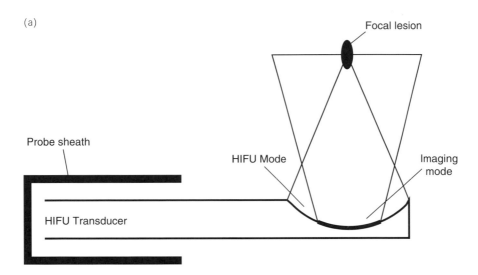

(b)

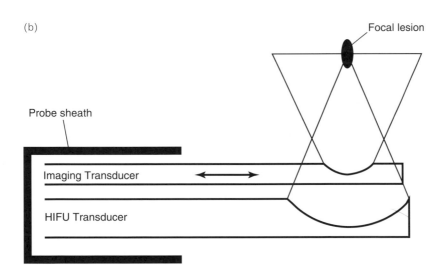

Fig. 12.6. Transrectal HIFU systems. (a) The same transducer operating at 4.0 MHz is used for imaging and therapy (Sonablate, Focal Surgery, Inc., Milpitas, USA). (b) In this device two separate transducers for imaging and therapy are incorporated in a transrectal probe sheath (Ablatherm, Technomed International, Lyon, France).[24,36] (c) (next page) By moving the HIFU focus under computer control in a longitudinal (sagittal view, left) and transverse (transverse view, right) plane, a clinically useful lesion volume is generated. UT, high-intensity focused ultrasound transducer; FZ, focal zone; VL, volume of lesion; P, prostate; U, urethra. (Adapted from ref. 23.)

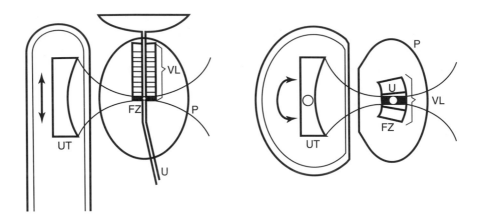

Fig. 12.6 (c)

with a plano-concave spherical lens.[18,19] The focal length was in the range of 15–18 cm and the site intensity used was approximately 1000 W/cm^2. Despite encouraging results this approach was not introduced into clinical routine, in particular because of the long treatment time (up to 8 h) and the fact that the cranium had to be removed for therapy, as HIFU does not penetrate bony structures.

Most of the HIFU devices currently being used for clinical trials damage an ellipsoidal tissue volume that is approximately 2 mm in diameter and 10 mm long. In order to create a clinically useful tissue volume, a multiplicity of laterally or axially displaced individual lesions are generated by physical movement of the sound head or by electronically sweeping the focused beam, as exemplified in Fig. 12.6c for a transrectal device.[17,21–24]

By far the greatest body of clinical experience with extracorporeal HIFU is currently in the field of ophthalmology for the treatment of glaucoma.[25,26] The transducer used has a focal length of 90 mm and operates with a frequency of 4.6 MHz; the focal lesion has a length of 3.0 mm and a width of 0.4 mm. The transducer is coupled to the eye with a sterile, saline-filled water bath, similar to that used in immersion ultrasonography. Using the aiming light and the confocal A scan, the focal zone is directed towards the target area.

Within the past 20 years, several research groups have developed extracorporeal HIFU devices and detailed mathematical calculations on this technology are available, yet results of human trials using these systems are not yet available.[27–29] It is beyond the scope of this chapter to describe all these instruments. Recently, Ioritani et al[30] reported on a novel extracorporeal device. The ultrasound source is a spherical piezoceramic (diameter 100 mm, curvature 120 mm) operating at 1.65 MHz. The maximum site intensity at the focal point was 4200 W/cm^2. Histological analyses of treated areas (canine thigh muscle, kidney and prostate) revealed sharply delineated coagulative necrosis within the focal area. This area was surrounded by a thin annular zone (0.5–1 mm) with massive deformity of the tissue structure. Outside this zone, bleeding or other tissue changes were not observed. These histological data indicate that the therapeutic effect of this system is most likely to be a combination of thermal effects (centre zone) and tissue cavitation (intermediate zone).

Experimental studies

The numerous animal studies evaluating the therapeutic effect of HIFU reported over the past 40 years can be divided into two groups—those evaluating the impact on naïve organs and those assessing the effect on experimental tumours. The second group are reviewed in Chapter 10; this chapter, therefore, concentrates on the former group, with particular reference to urology. In non-urological organs, the histological impact of HIFU has been extensively studied in brain, liver, eye and soft tissue (such as thigh muscle).[31–34]

In the field of urology, experimental data regarding kidney, bladder and prostate are available.[21,24,35,36] As Chapter 10 describes the application for bladder tumours, this issue is not discussed herein.

Chapelon et al[35] determined the histological impact on 124 rat and 16 canine kidneys with 1 MHz (site intensity 2750 W/cm^2) and 2.25 MHz (site intensity 3200 W/cm^2) HIFU transducer.[5] Rat kidneys were treated after externalization outside the abdominal cavity. The largest and best-focused lesions were achieved with an exposure period of 200 ms and a site intensity of 3200 W/cm^2 (2.25 MHz). Subsequently, canine kidneys were treated transcutaneously. A kidney lesion was present in 63% of animals; macroscopically, lesions appeared as areas of renal infarction and histology revealed complete coagulation necrosis. Aiming accuracy was relatively poor, as the spleen was touched eight times, the left colon three times and lung and pancreas once. Furthermore, HIFU performed with high energy levels resulted in significant cutaneous burns in six dogs.

Using transrectal instrumentation that is currently used in human trials, Foster et al[21] studied the histological impact of HIFU on the prostates of 26 dogs that were killed 2 h to 12 weeks following treatment. Intraprostatic coagulative necrosis was consistently present. After 14 days, the early stages of cystic cavities were identified and, within 3 months, cystic cavities had formed. In all animals, surrounding and intervening structures such as the rectal wall and the prostate capsule were intact. A similar study was conducted by Gelet et al[24] on 37 beagles. An intraprostatic coagulative necrosis was present in the vast majority of animals; this subsequently formed a cystic cavity after 4 weeks. Both studies demonstrate the feasibility and safety of prostatic tissue ablation via the transrectal route.

For both devices, clinical data concerning patients with BPH and localized prostate cancer are available.

Thus, HIFU applied extracorporeally or transrectally is capable of inducing precise, controllable contact- and irradiation-free in-depth tissue destruction. From these studies it is clear that HIFU is highly attractive as a minimally invasive therapy for benign tumours, such as BPH, but even more for cancer located in organs accessible to ultrasound.

The potential use of HIFU for oncological indications raises the important issue of whether HIFU treatment retards or accelerates the formation of distant metastases. In various studies no such evidence has been reported, apart from a report by Fry et al.[37] In their series an inexplicable increased rate of metastasis was found in animals treated with HIFU or chemotherapy, compared with the control group. It has been speculated that this was attributable to other factors, such as vigorous manipulation of the animals, rather than to HIFU or chemotherapy itself. Chapelon et al[38] determined the impact of HIFU on the development of tumour metastases of experimental prostate cancer. In the control population, 28% of animals developed distant metastases, whereas in HIFU-treated animals this percentage dropped to 16%.

From these data and the results of other studies it can be concluded that HIFU applied to cancer tissue does not accelerate the development of distant metastases; in fact, numerous studies have indicated that HIFU treatment reduces the rate of metastases.[39]

Human trials

Although the first clinical HIFU trials were reported at the beginning of the 1960s, broad clinical testing of this technology has only been reported in the field of ophthalmology. In a recent multicentre trial the therapeutic effect of HIFU in glaucoma refractory to conventional medical and surgical therapy was demonstrated.[25]

Whereas, before 1990, extraurological organs, such as the brain and eye, were the chief targets of investigation, major interest has been directed over the past 4 or 5 years to the field of urology, and particularly to the prostate. The recent development of compact HIFU transducer systems has been the technical basis for the development of transrectal devices enabling precise and safe prostatic tissue ablation.

HIFU-induced intraprostatic histological changes

At the authors' institution a total of 54 prostates were treated with transrectal HIFU prior to surgical removal.[23,40,41] All prostates were analysed histologically using whole-mount prostatic sections as described in detail previously.[23,40] Mapping of intraprostatic coagulative necrosis was possible in all specimens. As early as 1 h after HIFU, intraprostatic necrosis was demonstrable. Epithelial cells exhibited dark-staining pyknotic nuclei, with the surrounding cytoplasm being narrow and irregularly vacuolated (Fig. 12.7a). The epithelium was detached from the basal membrane and single cells were dissociated. Electron microscopy of fresh lesions (2–3 h after HIFU) revealed marked changes at the subcellular level.[40] After 7 days the target area was seen as a zone of classic haemorrhagic necrosis (Fig. 12.7b). Within 10 weeks, the coagulative necrosis was resorbed by granulation tissue rich in macrophages and capillary sprouts and a scar was formed (Fig. 12.7c).[40] The border between HIFU-treated and untreated tissue was extremely sharp, comprising only five to seven cell layers.[23] Thermolesions to intervening tissues were never observed, underlining the safety of the applied system. Using the second transrectal HIFU system currently available, Gelet et al[36] recently described the effect of HIFU on the histology of the human prostate, using a comparable study design. Patients were subjected to prostatectomy 2–48 h after HIFU. Whereas only minimal, if any, tissue effects were observed in patients in whom site intensities were lower than, or comparable to, those in canine trials, well-defined coagulative necrosis was consistently present in patients treated with higher site intensities. These segments were rectangular and their dimensions were equal to, or slightly greater than, the theoretical target volume. Side effects were only minimal. Both series demonstrate that transrectal HIFU enables precise, predictable and safe intraprostatic tissue ablation.

Transrectal HIFU for BPH

An international clinical trial was initiated in June 1992 to evaluate the safety and efficacy of transrectal HIFU for BPH. In this non-randomized Phase II clinical trial, approximately 250 BPH patients have been treated, worldwide, with a transrectal device.[22,23,42] The clinical data, reported here, of the authors' series of 86 patients, correlate well with those reported by others.[22,23,42] Significant clinical improvements were observed both in the subjective [American Urological Association (AUA) score, quality of life] and objective (uroflow, residual volume) BPH parameters (Fig. 12.8). After 12 months, the Q_{max} improved by 47% and the subjective symptoms were reduced by a mean of 55%. A reduction of the AUA symptom score by more than 50% was noted in 77% of patients (Fig. 12.8). Intraprostatic cystic cavities, comparable to those after transurethral resection of the prostate, were demonstrable by transrectal ultrasonography (7.5 MHz) in approximately 25% of patients.[23] Overall, HIFU treatment was well tolerated. Rectoscopy immediately after the procedure revealed normal results in all patients.[23] The predominant side effect, observed in almost all patients, was urinary retention. For this reason a 10 Fr cystostomy catheter was routinely placed intraoperatively, and was removed on an outpatient

(a)

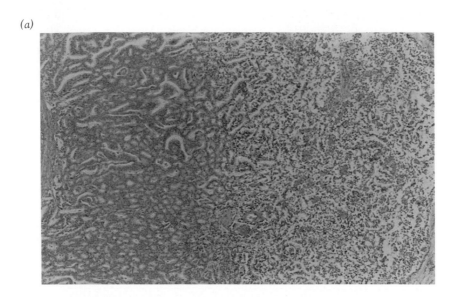

(b)

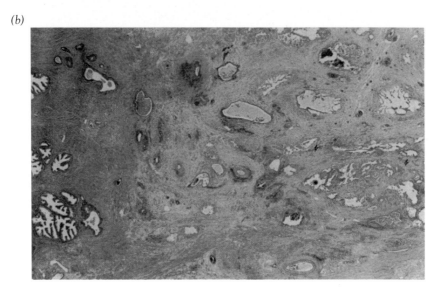

Fig. 12.7. Time course of HIFU-induced intraprostatic changes. (a) 3 h after HIFU: an area of prostate cancer is shown. The fresh HIFU necrosis (right) is characterized by pale staining, hyperchromatic nuclei and detachment of epithelial cells from the basement membrane. The darkly stained vital tissue is located to the left. (b) 7 days after HIFU: the HIFU-induced haemorrhagic intraprostatic necrosis is characterized by loss of the glandular lining and the presence of erythrocytes within the connective tissue. (c) (opposite) 10 weeks after HIFU: the HIFU-induced coagulative necrosis is organized to a fibrotic scar. Note the clear demarcation of the viable tissue (right) and the fibrotic scar (left). On the far left, remnants of glandular tissue can be seen.

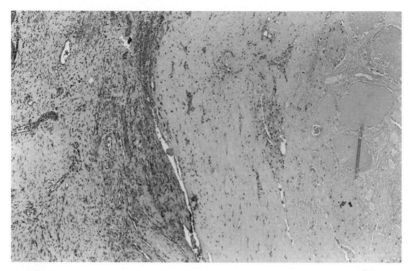

Fig. 12.7 (c)

basis after a mean of 6 days. The majority of sexually active patients reported haematospermia, which disappeared spontaneously after 4–6 weeks.

These data demonstrate that transrectal HIFU is capable of improving subjective and objective BPH parameters. The major advantage of

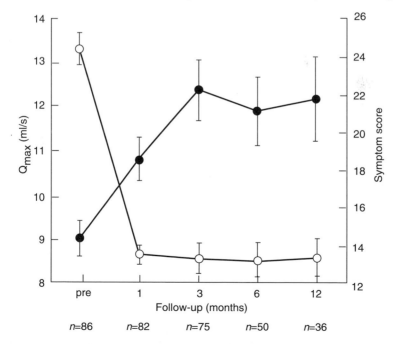

Fig. 12.8. Improvement of Q_{max} (●) and AUA symptom score (○) after transrectal HIFU for symptomatic BPH. Both parameters improve significantly after transrectal HIFU. Follow-up data (1 year) demonstrate a prolonged therapeutic effect.

transrectal HIFU is its ability to induce contact-free intraprostatic necrosis, thus avoiding urethral manipulation. Consequently, postoperative dysuria and urethral discomfort are almost absent and, in theory, the risk of urethral strictures should be minimal.[22,23] Currently the HIFU procedure for BPH is undergoing significant technical improvements, such as increased intraprostatic lesion volume and enhanced energy deposit at the bladder neck.

Transrectal HIFU for localized prostate cancer

The ability to ablate intraprostatic tissue without contact or irradiation makes HIFU even more attractive as a minimally invasive treatment option for localized prostate cancer (PC). Before any clinical application, the histological impact of HIFU on PC needs to be evaluated carefully. The authors therefore targeted HIFU ultrasound guided on clearly visible hypoechoic and palpable histology-proven PC (T_{2a} and T_{2b}) prior to radical prostatectomy.[41] Aiming accuracy was excellent. In all cases (n=10) the PC was correctly targeted: in two cases, the entire PC was destroyed by HIFU; in the remaining eight, a mean of 53% of the cancer was destroyed (range 37–78%). With a maximum length of the treatment zone of about 4 cm, 15–20 cm^3 prostatic tissue can be reliably ablated within a treatment time of 90–120 min. These histological data indicate that transrectal HIFU is an attractive, novel, minimally invasive treatment option for localized PC and preliminary clinical data are already available. Gelet et al[43] treated eight PC patients at clinical stages A (n=1) and B (n=7). HIFU therapy involved the whole prostate in one or two sessions. Five patients have completed a 2 month follow-up: in four, prostate-specific antigen (PSA) was normal and biopsies negative; one patient was found to have residual cancer and was treated by orchiectomy. Side effects were spontaneously healing rectal burns (n=2), rectourethral fistula (n=1) and periprostatic urinary extravasation (n=1). At the authors' institution, five patients with localized PC have been treated so far, with minimal postoperative morbidity. After 3 months, four of these patients had negative biopsies and a serum PSA within the normal range. These preliminary data indicate that transrectal HIFU achieves local tumour destruction and could therefore ultimately become a minimally invasive therapeutic option for localized PC.

Testis

Recently, the histological impact of transcutaneous HIFU on the human testis was reported.[44] Testes of patients with metastatic prostatic cancer (n=4) undergoing scrotal orchiectomy were exposed to therapeutic transcutaneous HIFU (frequency 4.0 MHz, site intensity 1680 W/cm^2) immediately before surgery. Histologically, ablated testicular tissue exhibited definite signs of necrosis with detachment of germinal epithelium, shrinking of nuclei and cell disintegration. On the basis of these histological findings, a clinical trial evaluating this novel approach has been initiated.[44]

HIFU and the immune system

Although this field is very speculative, recent studies evaluating this interesting aspect warrant a brief mention. In BPH tissue obtained 4–12 weeks after transrectal HIFU, a significant increase in activation marker expression is present, as recently shown in the authors' laboratory. These data indicate that HIFU induces an influx primarily of $CD4^+$ peripheral cells. Of particular interest is the immune status after HIFU of cancer cells and preliminary data regarding this issue are available. Yang et al[45] demonstrated that tumour growth following a second tumour challenge in previously HIFU-cured animals was significantly reduced. Similar data were reported by Wagai et al,[46] who demonstrated that rats bearing the Horie's sarcoma curatively treated with HIFU ($1000 \ W/cm^2$) developed a high resistance to subsequent tumour challenge. These effects may be related to enhanced antitumour immune activity. It has been speculated that tumour breakdown products after HIFU treatment may enhance tumour immunogenicity and augment host immunity. These observations are particularly important for oncological applications, as there is the risk of tumour cells surviving after HIFU therapy, owing to multifocal distribution, location of tumour cells at the border of the treatment zone and micrometastases.

Conclusions and future perspectives

Ultrasound therapy using purely the mechanical effect is in routine clinical use for endoscopic contact lithotripsy, ultrasonic tissue aspiration and non-contact ESWL. Extracorporeal ultrasonic tissue tripsy is a novel technique based on the generation of high-frequency shock waves permitting extracorporeal application and the lesioning of deep structures, due to the long focal length. The major disadvantage of this approach is the fact that the predominant therapeutic effect is cavitation, which leads to rather uncontrolled tissue ablation.

Monocrystal HIFU devices permit precise tissue destruction without damage to adjacent structures. Currently, the broader clinical application of this technique is hindered by the fairly short focal length available. This limits the clinical application to superficial regions, such as prostatic tissue using the transrectal approach.

In the near future, various technical innovations regarding HIFU therapy are expected to revolutionize its clinical application. The most important step in this direction would be the availability of a phased-array transducer of variable focal length (Fig. 12.9)[47]. Once these transducers are to hand, it will

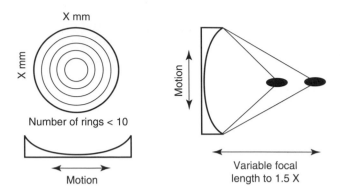

Fig. 12.9. Theoretical model for an annular phased-array HIFU transducer. In this theoretical model, a number of annular piezoceramic elements are mounted on a concave disc permitting individual adaptation of the focal length. Electronic HIFU focusing is combined with mechanical beam steering. Disadvantages of this approach are slow imaging and sophisticated multiple channel electronics.

be possible to delimit the target zone in two planes on the computer screen and the area in question will be precisely ablated. In addition, longer focal lengths are urgently required to facilitate in-depth tissue destruction and an extracorporeal approach. The availability of varying focal sizes and shorter duty cycles would help to reduce treatment time, which is important in the context of anaesthesia requirement. Finally, the incorporation of MRI equipment permits better visualization of the target tissue, of temperature changes and of the effects of treatment. In experimental settings, this approach has already yielded encouraging data.[48]

Thus, the ultimate objective for clinical HIFU is as a form of non-invasive, transcutaneous, ultrasound- or MRI-guided anticancer treatment, for both curative and palliative purposes.

References

1. Driller J, Lizzi F L. Therapeutic application of ultrasound: a review. IEEE 1987; 12: 33–40
2. Barnett S B, Ter Haar G R, Ziskin M C et al. Current status of research on biophysical effects of ultrasound. Ultrasound Med Biol 1994; 20: 205–218
3. Marberger M. Disintegration of renal and ureteral calculi with ultrasound. Urol Clin North Am 1983; 10: 729–742
4. Krawitt D R, Addonizio J C. Ultrasonic aspiration of prostate, bladder tumors, and stones. Urology 1987; 30: 579–580
5. Chopp R T, Shah B B, Addonizio J C. Use of ultrasonic surgical aspirator in renal surgery. Urology 1983; 22: 157–159
6. Hodgson W J B, DelGuercio L R M. Preliminary experience in liver surgery using the ultrasonic scalpel. Surgery 1984; 2: 230–234
7. Ishibashi K, Shiozawa H, Tochimoto M et al. Endoscopic ultrasonic aspirator and its clinical application. Jpn J Endourol ESWL 1994; 7: 298
8. Chaussy C, Schmiedt E, Jocham D et al. First clinical experience with extracorporeally induced destruction of kidney stones by shock waves. J Urol 1982; 127: 417–420
9. Jenkins A D. Extracorporeal shock wave lithotripsy of renal stones. In: Marberger M, Fitzpatrick J M, Jenkins A D, Pak C Y C (eds) Stone surgery. Edinburgh: Churchill Livingstone, 1991; 15–47

10. Marberger M, Türk C, Steinkogler I. Painless piezoelectric extracorporeal lithotripsy. J Urol 1988; 139; 695–699
11. Russo P, Mies C, Huryk R et al. Histopathologic and ultrastructural correlates of tumor growth suppression by high energy shock waves. J Urol 1987; 137: 338–342
12. Oosterhof G O N, Smits G A H, de Ruyter A N. In vivo effect of high energy shock waves on urological tumors: an evaluation of treatment modalities. J Urol 1990; 144: 785–798
13. Vallancien G, Chartier-Kastler E, Chopin D et al. Focused extracorporeal pyrotherapy: experimental results. Eur Urol 1991; 20: 211–219
14. Vallancien G, Harouni M, Veillon B et al. extracorporeal pyrotherapy: feasibility study in man. J Endourol 1992; 6: 173–181
15. Vallancien G, Chartier-Kastler E, Bataille N et al. Focused extracorporeal pyrotherapy. Eur Urol 1993; 23(suppl 1): 48–52
16. Fry F J. Intense focused ultrasound in medicine. Eur Urol 1993; 23(suppl 1): 2–7
17. Ter Haar G. Focused ultrasound therapy. Curr Opinion Urol 1994; 4: 89–92
18. Fry W J, Barnard J W, Fry F J et al. Ultrasonic lesions in the mammalian central nervous system. Science 1955; 122: 517–518
19. Meyers R, Fry W J, Fry F J et al. Early experiences with ultrasonic irradiation of the pallidofugal and nigral complexes in hyperkinetic and hypertonic disorders. J Neurosurg 1959; 16: 32–54
20. Ter Haar G, Sinnett D, Rivens I. High intensity focused ultrasound—a surgical technique for the treatment of discrete liver tumors. Phys Med Biol 1989; 34: 1743–1750
21. Foster R S, Bihrle R, Sanghvi N T et al. Production of prostatic lesions in canines using transrectally administered high intensity focused ultrasound. Eur Urol 1993; 23: 330–336
22. Bihrle R, Foster R S, Sanghvi N T et al. High intensity focused ultrasound for the treatment of BPH: early US clinical experience. J Urol 1994; 151: 1271–1275
23. Madersbacher S, Kratzik C, Susani M, Marberger M. Treatment of benign prostatic hyperplasia with high intensity focused ultrasound. J Urol 1994; 152: 1956–1961
24. Gelet A, Chapelon J Y, Margonari J et al. Prostatic tissue destruction by high intensity focused ultrasound: experimentation on canine prostate. J Endourol 1993; 7: 249–253
25. Silvermann R H, Vogelsang B, Rondeau M J, Coleman D J. Therapeutic ultrasound for the treatment of glaucoma. Am J Ophthalmol 1991; 111: 327–337
26. Lizzi F L. High-precision thermotherapy for small lesions. Eur Urol 1993; 23(suppl 1): 23–28
27. Vaughan M G, Ter Haar G R, Hill C R et al. Minimally invasive cancer surgery using focused ultrasound: a pre-clinical, normal tissue study. Br J Radiol 1994; 67: 267–274
28. Linke C A, Carstensen E L, Frizzell L A et al. Localized tissue destruction by high-intensity focused ultrasound. Arch Surg 1973; 107: 887–891
29. Hill C R, Rivens I, Vaughan M G, Ter Haar G T. Lesion development in focused ultrasound surgery: a general model. Ultrasound Med Biol 1994; 20: 259–269
30. Ioritani N, Sirai S, Taguchi K et al. Effects of high intensity ultrasound heating on the normal and cancer tissue. Jpn J Endourol ESWL 1994; 7: 299
31. Chen L, Rivens T, Ter Haar G R et al. Histological changes in rat liver tumours treated with high intensity focused ultrasound. Ultrasound Med Biol 1993; 19: 67–74
32. Hynynen K. The threshold for thermally significant cavitation in dog's thigh muscle in vivo. Ultrasound Med Biol 1991; 17: 157–169
33. Rutzen A R, Roberts C W, Driller J et al. Production of corneal lesions using high-intensity focused ultrasound. Cornea 1990; 9: 324–330
34. Yang R, Sanghvi N T, Rescorla F J et al. Extracorporeal liver ablation using sonography-guided high-intensity focused ultrasound. Invest Radiol 1992; 27: 796–803
35. Chapelon J Y, Margonari J, Theillere Y et al. Effects of high-energy focused ultrasound on kidney tissue in the rat and the dog. Eur Urol 1992; 22: 147–152
36. Gelet A, Chapelon J Y, Margonari J et al. High intensity focused ultrasound experimentation on human benign prostatic hypertrophy. Eur Urol 1993; 23(suppl 1): 44–47
37. Fry F J, Johnson L K. Tumor irradiation with intense ultrasound. Ultrasound Med Biol 1978; 4: 337–341
38. Chapelon J Y, Margonari J, Vernier F et al. In vivo effects of high-intensity ultrasound on prostatic adenocarcinoma Dunning R3327. Cancer Res 1992; 52: 6353–6357
39. Yang R, Sanghvi N T, Rescorla F J et al. Liver cancer ablation with extracorporeal high-intensity focused ultrasound. Eur Urol 1993; 23(suppl 1): 17–22

40. Susani M, Madersbacher S, Kratzik C et al. Morphology of tissue destruction induced by focused ultrasound. Eur Urol 1993: 23(suppl 1): 34–38
41. Marberger M, Susani M, Madersbacher S et al. Effect of high intensity focused ultrasound on human prostate cancer. J Urol 1994; 151(suppl): 436A
42. Ebert T, Miller S, Schmitz-Draeger B, Ackermann R. High intensity focused ultrasound (HIFU) in patients with benign prostatic hyperplasia. J Urol 1994; 151(suppl): 399A
43. Gelet A, Chapelon J Y, Bouvier R et al. Treatment of localized prostatic cancer by high intensity focused ultrasound (HIFU) delivered by transrectal route: preliminary results. 11th EAU Congr 1994; 267A
44. Kratzik C, Madersbacher S, Susani M, Marberger M. Percutaneous application of high intensity focused ultrasound in urology. Proc 23rd SIU Congr, Sydney 1994; 76
45. Yang R, Reilly C R, Rescorla F J et al. Effects of high-intensity focused ultrasound in the treatment of experimental neuroblastoma. J Pediatr Surg 1992; 27: 246–251
46. Wagai T, Kakata K, Mizuno S. Medical application of intense ultrasound. III. Destruction of malignant tumor by intense focused ultrasound. Annual report (1970). Tokyo: Medical Ultrasound Research Centre Tokyo, Jutendo University School of Medicine 1971; 35–39
47 Zanelli C L, Hennige C W, Sanghui N T. Design and characterization of a 10 cm annular array transducer for high intensity focused ultrasound (HIFU) applications. UFFC 1994
48. Hynynen K, Darkazanli A, Damianou C A et al. Tissue thermometry during ultrasound exposure. Eur Urol 1993; 23(suppl 1): 12–16

Contact Nd:YAG laser-assisted vasal anastomosis: clinical experience in 206 patients

13

Y.-H. Cho   S. W. Kim   J. H. Kim   M. S. Yoon

Introduction

Vasectomy has been one of the most commonly performed operations in Korea over the past two decades. Subsequently, the frequency of vasovasostomy has increased dramatically because many of these vasectomized men desire to regain their fertility. Common reasons cited include divorce with remarriage, loss of a child, improved financial status and altered attitude toward family size.

Currently, the most widely used method for obtaining an accurate vasal anastomosis is the microsurgical technique described by Silber.[1] However, this procedure requires special microsurgical training and long operative times. Recently, the application of lasers to medicine has been expanded rapidly. Laser-assisted vasal anastomosis was described first by Lynne et al[2] in animal models in 1983 and the use of lasers, mainly carbon dioxide (CO_2) or neodymium:yttrium aluminium garnet (Nd:YAG), has been explored widely by several surgeons in search of a rapid and simple technique for vasal anastomosis.[3,4] Their positive results encouraged the authors to introduce contact Nd:YAG laser-assisted vasovasostomy (CLAVA) to clinical practice following an experimental study in dogs utilizing the laser.[5] CLAVA is a simplified surgical technique that the average practising urologist can perform rapidly with minimal complications and acceptable results.

The authors' clinical experience obtained from 206 patients is presented.

Patients and methods

Between February 1992 and March 1993, 206 patients underwent CLAVA in the authors' department. All surgical procedures were performed in the operating room under local anaesthesia as described by Kaye et al[6] and patients were discharged from the unit on the following day.

Beginning with a midline scrotal incision, the vas was identified and dissected from surrounding scar tissue. The vas was subsequently transected at an appropriate distance to free both ends with a cold knife. After the open ends of the vas had been gently dilated with vas dilators, specimens of vas fluid were taken from the proximal ends and submitted for examination for the presence or absence of sperm. A 26 gauge needle was used as an intraluminal stent for all vasal anastomoses.

Four full-thickness sutures through the mucosa and serosa of the vas were placed at the 3, 6, 9 and 12 o'clock positions using Prolene 7/0 before the use of the laser. Four sutures were sufficient for most patients, but if there was marked dilatation of the proximal vas, another suture was necessary to decrease the size discrepancy and facilitate welding. These sutures were placed for traction to assist in the initial approximation and secured the welded seam of the anastomosis after laser treatment (Fig. 13.1). Complete haemostasis and meticulous drying of the operation site were achieved before the laser-assisted anastomosis.

A contact Nd:YAG laser (SLT Japan Co., Ltd, Tokyo, Japan), wavelength 1064 nm, was used. The opposed tissue edges were welded together by a synthetic sapphire probe (ERP4) which, by foot pedal control, emitted pulses of 2.0 s duration and 5 W power, 250–300 J, for unilateral CLAVA without a microscope. The visible endpoint of laser application was tissue coaptation and light brown discoloration without charring or blackening. The scrotal skin was closed in two-layer fashion with 4/0 chromic sutures.

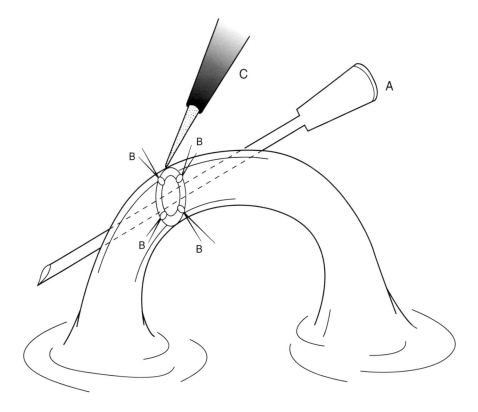

Fig. 13.1. Technique for contact Nd:YAG laser-assisted vasal anastomosis. A, stenting with 26 gauge needle; B, four full-thickness Prolene 7/0 stay sutures at the 3, 6, 9 and 12 o'clock positions; C, welding the apposed tissue edges by means of the contact laser.

The time required for the achievement of a unilateral CLAVA averaged 5 min and the entire operative time was 70 min. Sperm counts were performed in week 6 and pregnancy analyses were obtained 6–13 months after CLAVA.

Results

The ages of patients ranged from 28 to 50 years (average 38 years). Common reasons for CLAVA included altered attitude toward family size (140/206, 68%), divorce with remarriage (39/206, 19%), psychological inability to cope with impotence (11/206, 5%), failure of previous conventional vasovasostomy (10/206, 5%) and loss of a child (6/206, 3%).

Of the total 206 patients, 153 and 84 had patency and pregnancy rates evaluated in week 6 and 6–13 months after CLAVA, respectively, according to the duration of vas obstruction, the levels of CLAVA and the status of spermatic fluid leakage. The results, detailed in Tables 13.1 and 13.2, showed that patency and pregnancy rates were higher for those in whom vasectomy had taken place less than 5 years previously, in whom the anastomosis involved bilateral straight vas to straight vas and in whom there was leakage of spermatic fluid than in those with an obstructive interval of more than 5 years, with any anastomosis involving the convoluted portion of the vas and with no spermatic fluid leakage.

The overall success rate for patency on week 6 after CLAVA was 92% (140/153), and for pregnancy 6–13 months after CLAVA was 39% (33/84).

Parameter	No. of patients	Patency (%)†
Obstructive interval of vas		
< 5 years	52	50 (96)
5–10 years	80	73 (91)
> 10 years	21	17 (81)
Level of CLAVA‡		
Bilateral st. vas to st. vas	112	105 (94)
St. vas to st. vas and st. vas to con. vas	31	27 (87)
Bilateral st. vas to con. vas	10	8 (80)
Spermatic fluid leakage		
Bilateral	89	84 (94)
Unilateral	32	30 (94)
None	32	26 (81)

Table 13.1. Patency rate* of 153 evaluable patients from a total of 206 undergoing contact Nd:YAG laser-assisted vasovasostomy (CLAVA)

*Overall patency rate 92% (140/153); †followed up on week 6 after CLAVA; ‡st., straight; con., convoluted.

Parameter	No. of patients	Pregnancy (%)†
Obstructive interval of vas		
<5 years	36	15 (42)
5–10 years	39	16 (41)
>10 years	9	2 (22)
Level of CLAVA‡		
Bilateral st. vas to st. vas	62	28 (42)
St. vas to st. vas and st. vas to con. vas	12	3 (25)
Bilateral st. vas to con. vas	10	2 (20)
Spermatic fluid leakage		
Bilateral	55	23 (42)
Unilateral	15	6 (40)
None	14	4 (29)

Table 13.2. Pregnancy rate* of 84 evaluable patients from a total of 206 undergoing CLAVA
*Overall pregnancy rate 39% (33/84); †followed up 6 and 13 months after CLAVA; ‡abbreviations as in Table 13.1.

Semen analysis on week 6 after CLAVA showed that the average ejaculate volume was 3.8 ml, with motility 38% and morphology 53% of normal form, sperm density equal to or more than 20×10^6/ml in 58% (81/140) and less than 20×10^6/ml in 42% (59/140).

In all 206 cases, there was no significant complication, sperm granuloma, or even significant swelling or haematoma after CLAVA.

Discussion

Microsurgical anastomosis is the most common technique currently used for vasovasostomies. Patency rates vary and appear to be related to the skill of the surgeon, the frequency of performing each procedure, and the type of suture material involved.[7,8] Any method that standardized the procedure and provided uniform results would be desirable, and is potentially feasible with laser welding. Unlike the conventional microsurgical suture technique, laser vasal anastomosis does not demand any special manual skill or training of the surgeon.

Several recent studies have shown that patency and pregnancy rates in laser-assisted vasal anastomosis are the same as those for the conventional microsurgical technique.[3,4]

Although the CO_2, argon and Nd:YAG lasers have all been used successfully to anastomose various structures, the most popular type of laser for vasal anastomosis is the CO_2 or Nd:YAG laser. However, in the non-contact laser which uses a 'joystick' (handpiece), welding of the vas is achieved by the back-and-forth movement of an energy beam.[9] In focusing the beam, the power density is lowered by a factor that varies inversely with the square of the radius of the spot. The result is that evaporation is slower, resulting in a thicker zone of thermal damage due to heat conduction from the surface of the wound.[10]

In the study described here, a contact Nd:YAG laser using a synthetic sapphire probe was used in welding of the vas to avoid defocusing and to apply the laser energy evenly to the tissue. Contact probes work only when in direct contact with the tissue. Originally, a contact sapphire probe was introduced to permit precise cutting of soft tissue, with excellent first-pass haemostasis of transected vessels but without the extensive thermal damage characteristic of Nd:YAG beams delivered by non-contact fibres. In addition, whereas approximately 30–40% of the beam energy can be lost to backscatter in the non-contact Nd:YAG laser, energy loss to backscatter is cut to less than 5% in the contact Nd:YAG laser, and the overall laser output needed to achieve a given therapeutic effect is 75–90% less than would be needed in a non-contact procedure.[11,12]

More than 59 types (in terms of shape and diameter) of contact sapphire probes have been developed so far. In this study, a sapphire probe with a diameter of 0.4 mm (Frosted Laser Scalpels, ERP4; SLT Japan Co., Ltd) was used and a temperature of 60–65°C was maintained. This temperature enables protein coagulation to take place without tissue vaporization.[13]

Successful vasovasostomy is required for accurate anastomosis of the two ends of the vas deferens. The authors therefore used a 26 gauge needle as an intraluminal stent to approximate accurately, to suture and to avoid post-operative narrowing or occlusion of the anastomosis site. In the preliminary study, the dog was used as animal model because it has internal genital organs of size and diameter similar to those in humans. To investigate the optimum level of power of the contact Nd:YAG laser in vasal anastomosis, 3, 4, 5, 6, 7 and 8 W power levels were tested: 5 W appeared to be the most appropriate in terms of speed, economy of energy and welding without carbonization.[5]

As a laser application method, rather than a continuous wave, 2.0 s pulses were used. Pulsing the laser in short bursts enables the maximum power output of the laser to be used without concern of excessive damage.[9]

These results have demonstrated the feasibility of this simple surgical procedure with an acceptable success rate in sterilized men. This is a very rapid procedure compared with a suture technique. For the 206 patients, the mean operation time was 70 min. The overall patency rate of 92% is similar to that for conventional microsurgical anastomosis, although follow-up was less than 2 months in most patients.[14,15] With regard to the pregnancy success rate, despite the relatively short-term follow-up (6–13 months after CLAVA) the rate of 39% was acceptable in comparison with the pregnancy rates achieved with conventional microsurgical techniques.[16,17]

There was no significant complication, sperm granuloma, or even significant swelling or haematoma in any treated patient. There is no question that more experience and longer follow-up periods are required to judge this type of surgery adequately.

In conclusion, CLAVA is at least equal to conventional microsurgical techniques in success rates and is definitely easier to perform surgically.

References

1. Silber S J. Vasectomy and vasectomy reversal. Fertil Steril 1978; 29: 125–140
2. Lynne C M, Carter M, Morris J et al. Laser assisted vas anastomosis: a preliminary report. Lasers Surg Med 1983; 3: 261–263
3. Shanberg A, Tansey L, Baghdassarian R et al. Laser-assisted vasectomy reversal: experience in 32 patients. J Urol 1990; 143: 528–530
4. Samuel K R. Further clinical experience with CO_2 laser in microsurgical vasovasostomy. Urology 1988; 32: 225–227
5. Cho Y H, Lee J Y, Hahn H G et al. Vasal anastomoses in dogs using contact neodymium: yttrium aluminium garnet (Nd:YAG) laser. Lasers Surg Med 1994; 15: 65–70
6. Kaye K W, Gonzalez R, Fraley E E. Microsurgical vasovasostomy: an outpatient procedure under local anesthesia. J Urol 1983; 129: 992–994
7. Shelor W C Jr, Witherington R. Comparison of polypropylene and polyglycolic acid suture in experimental vasovasostomy. Invest Urol 1975; 13: 223–226
8. Thomas A J, Pontes J E, Buddhdev H, Pierce J M. Vasovasostomy: evaluation of four surgical techniques. Fertil Steril 1979; 32: 324–328
9. Abstein G T, Joffe N S. Lasers in medicine, 2nd ed. London: Chapman & Hall, 1989; 2: 42–44
10. Fournier G R Jr. Laser surgery. In: Tanagho E A, McAninch J W (eds) Frontiers in Smith's general urology, 13th ed. London: Prentice Hall, 1991; 439–447
11. Daikuzono N, Joffe S N. Artificial sapphire probe for contact photocoagulation and tissue vaporization with Nd:YAG laser. Med Instrum 1985; 119: 173–178
12. Daikuzono N. Contact delivery systems and accessories. In: Joffe S N, Oguro Y (eds) Advances in Nd:YAG laser surgery. New York: Springer-Verlag, 1988; 19–29
13. Weiner P, Finkelstein L, Greene C H, Debias D A. Efficacy of the neodymium:YAG laser in vasovasostomy: a preliminary communication. Lasers Surg Med 1987; 6: 536–537
14. Willsher M K, Novicki D E. Simplified technique for microscopic vasovasostomy. Urology 1980; 15: 147–149
15. Fenster H, McLoughlin M G. Vasovasostomy: is the microscope necessary? Urology 1981; 18: 60–64
16. Cos L R, Valvo J R, Davis R S. Vasovasostomy: current state of the art. Urology 1983; 22: 6–7
17. Requeda E, Charron J, Roberts K. Fertilizing capacity and sperm antibodies in vasovasostomized men. Fertil Steril 1983; 39: 197–203

Laser dosimetry studies in the human prostate

14

J. N. Kabalin

Introduction

Laser prostatectomy has become a viable and popular treatment alternative for the management of bladder outlet obstruction due to benign prostatic hyperplasia (BPH).[1–8] To date, these procedures have primarily utilized the neodymium:yttrium aluminium garnet (Nd:YAG) laser wavelength to produce deep tissue coagulation followed by necrosis and subsequent slough of the obstructing prostatic transition zone, resulting in relief of voiding symptoms. The first free-beam side-firing Nd:YAG delivery fibre that could be used under direct vision through standard cystoscopic equipment to perform laser prostatectomy—the Urolase[TM]—was introduced in initial human clinical application in Australia in 1990.[1] This was followed by the first multicentre trials in the United States beginning in 1991.[2] Today, at least a dozen more-or-less dissimilar free-beam Nd:YAG laser delivery systems are available, with a variety of designs and laser beam output configurations. Unfortunately, until recently, little or no objective data have been available to support either the choice of power setting or the timing of laser applications to achieve optimal tissue ablation in the prostate, using any of these new delivery fibres. The author has previously reported efforts, first in a potato model and then in a canine prostate model, to define dosimetry curves for tissue ablation with the Urolase.[9] A model in vivo has now been developed, which is being used to extend these observations to the human prostate in an attempt to confirm and delineate optimal treatment parameters for laser prostatectomy using the Urolase and other fibre delivery systems in humans.

Patients and methods

Transurethral laser irradiation of the prostate was performed in 21 adult men with either peripheral zone prostate cancers (clinical stage B) or myoinvasive transitional cell carcinoma of the bladder (clinical stage B) immediately before planned radical prostatectomy or cystoprostatectomy. Patients with a previous history of prostatic surgery were excluded. Mean patient age was 65 years (range 47–71 years). At the time of radical cancer surgery and under the same general anaesthetic, patients were placed in the dorsal lithotomy position and prepared sterilely as for standard cystoscopy, which was performed using a 21 Fr cystoscope and sterile water irrigant at room temperature. A selected side-firing laser fibre was advanced into the prostatic urethra under direct vision and, using a standard Nd:YAG laser source capable of continuous output, laser irradiation was delivered at a single lateral spot location to one or both prostatic lateral lobes (3 o'clock and/or 9 o'clock) for variable treatment times at variable power settings as described below. In this fashion, overlap of laser-induced coagulation effects was minimized to allow careful postoperative measurements of each individual laser application site. All laser application times were continuous and without interruption. Following these brief laser applications, patients were repositioned and radical prostatectomy or cystoprostatectomy performed in the usual fashion. No external changes were observed in the prostate or surrounding pelvic tissues during open surgery following any laser treatment. Prostates were removed surgically, weighed and fixed overnight in formalin. Mean prostate weight in this series was 57 g (range 40–90 g). Cystoscopically, excess BPH tissue was estimated on average to be 23 g (range 10–45 g) and prostatic urethral length from bladder neck to verumontanum averaged 2.7 cm (range 2–4 cm).

At 24 h postoperatively, prostates were sectioned transversely. The area of transition zone coagulation was clearly visible in the gross specimens as a pale or white region (Fig. 14.1), and histological examination confirmed cellular coagulation injury corresponding to these gross observations. The zone of tissue coagulation produced by each individual laser application was measured in three dimensions, and results are reported both as the absolute depth of the lesion produced and as the volume of the lesion calculated from these measurements using the formula for a half-ellipsoid ($\pi/6 \times$ depth $\times$ width $\times$ length).

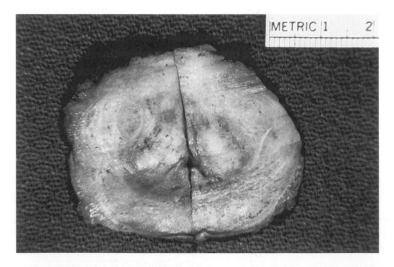

Fig. 14.1. Typical transverse section through a human radical prostatectomy specimen following bilateral lateral lobe irradiation with a Nd:YAG laser. The areas of transition zone coagulation are pale and demarcated by a rim of haemorrhage.

Utilizing this model for study in vivo of human prostatic laser dosimetry, complete quantitative dosimetry curves have been produced for two commonly used side-firing laser delivery fibres (see Table 14.1 for fibre specifications)—the ProLase II (Endocare, Inc., Irvine, CA, USA) and the Urolase (C.R. Bard, Inc., Covington, GA, USA).

Laser fibre delivery system	Core laser fibre (μm)	Laser reflecting mechanism	Maximum fibre diameter (Fr)	Beam angle of emission (degrees)	Beam divergence (degrees)
ProLase II (Endocare)	1000	Polished quartz	6.0	45 forward	35
Urolase (C.R. Bard)	600	Gold mirror	7.5	90 perpendicular	30

Table 14.1. Comparison of characteristics of two side-firing Nd:YAG laser delivery fibres currently in clinical use for coagulation prostatectomy

Results

Power dosimetry

Depth and volume of prostatic tissue ablation for single, continuous laser applications were measured at variable power settings from 20 to 80 W, while holding total energy delivery constant at 3600 J for each setting (Fig. 14.2). Peak tissue coagulation effects, both in terms of depth of tissue coagulation and total volume of tissue coagulation, were observed at the 40 W power setting for the Urolase fibre—up to a maximum of 14 mm depth of tissue penetration with a maximum volume of tissue coagulation of 4.23 cm^3. By comparison, the ProLase II fibre, with a slightly greater beam divergence (Table 14.1), larger spot size and resulting lower energy density laser applications, produced peak tissue coagulation effects at the 60 W power setting—up to a maximum of 13 mm depth of tissue penetration with a maximum volume of tissue coagulation of 3.92 cm^3. For both fibres, very high and very low power settings produced diminishing tissue effects, and optimal tissue coagulation was observed at mid-range power levels.

Time dosimetry

Holding the power setting constant at 40 W for the Urolase (this power setting having been observed with the Urolase fibre to produce the most efficient tissue coagulation in human prostates as described above), and constant at 60 W for the ProLase II (this power setting having been observed with the ProLase II fibre to produce the most efficient tissue coagulation), depth and volume of tissue coagulation were measured for variable treatment times between 45 and 120 s (Fig. 14.3). This implies

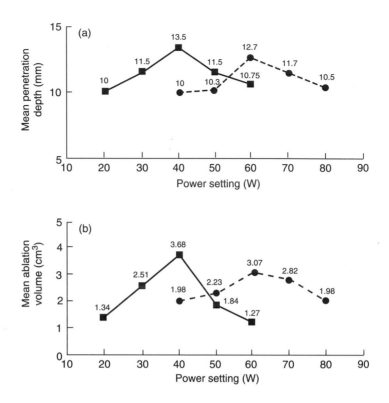

Fig. 14.2. *Dosimetry curves in the human prostate for variable power settings from 20 to 80 W, holding total energy delivery constant at 3600 J for each setting, for Urolase (■) and ProLase II (●) delivery systems, respectively. Mean values are shown above each curve. (a) Mean depth of tissue penetration for each power setting. (b) Mean volume of tissue coagulation for each power setting.*

variable energy delivery at either the 40 or 60 W power settings, respectively, which ranged from 2400 to 4800 J for each Urolase laser application and from 2700 to 5400 J for each ProLase II laser application. As the time of laser application was increased incrementally, the depth and also volume of tissue coagulation was observed to increase significantly up to 90 s with the Urolase and up to 60 s with the ProLase II. A plateau in tissue effects achieved was then observed for both delivery systems, with only small additional increases in tissue coagulation beyond approximately 90 s continuous laser application time at the 40 W power setting with the Urolase, and beyond approximately 60 s continuous laser application time at the 60 W power setting with the ProLase II.

Discussion

Clinical trials have demonstrated the safety and efficacy of Nd:YAG laser coagulation prostatectomy using a variety of delivery systems.[1–8,10–11]

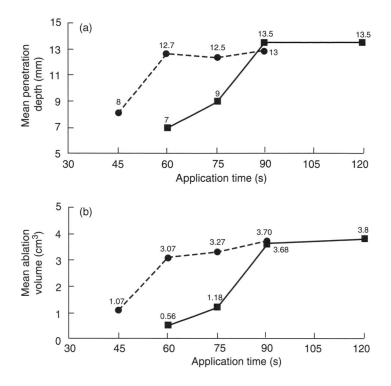

Fig. 14.3. Dosimetry curves in the human prostate for variable treatment times from 45 to 120 s, holding the power setting constant at 60 W for ProLase II (●) and constant at 40 W for Urolase (■) delivery systems, respectively. Mean values are shown above each curve. (a) Mean depth of tissue penetration for each treatment time. (b) Mean volume of tissue coagulation for each treatment time.

Work is in progress to maximize the efficacy of laser ablation of the prostate for the treatment of BPH.[9] For these efforts to prove successful, a better understanding is needed of the tissue effects produced in the human prostate by low energy density, relatively long duration Nd:YAG laser applications using the several laser delivery fibres now available. What all of these delivery systems have in common is their transurethral application and use of relatively large amounts of Nd:YAG laser energy to coagulate the obstructive transition zone of the prostate. However, operative techniques for laser coagulation prostatectomy are not yet standardized, in large part because of the wide variance in Nd:YAG laser beam configurations produced by the varying delivery fibres. For instance, the angle of incidence or emission of the beam from these fibres ranges from 45 to 105 degrees; the angle of divergence of the resultant laser beam varies between approximately 15 and 35 degrees. The latter parameter causes a significant variance in laser energy density and, potentially, of tissue effects produced by each device.

The ProLase II produces a laser beam emitted at a 45 degree angle forward from the device. The beam divergence is the widest of any fibre currently produced, at an angle of some 35 degrees. Unlike gold mirror devices, there is also considerable scatter of non-usable laser energy from the distal, polished quartz reflecting end of the fibre which can be easily demonstrated with a helium:neon aiming beam. Together, these features combine to produce the lowest energy density beam of any side-firing laser fibre currently available. The Urolase, using an external gold parabolic reflector, has a narrower angle of beam divergence at 30 degrees and none of the extraneous scatter of laser energy seen with the polished quartz internal reflector of the ProLase II. Thus, one would predict that the energy density of the laser beam output of the Urolase should be considerably greater than that of the ProLase II. The manufacturer, Endocare, states that the energy density of the ProLase II beam is approximately 55% that of the Urolase beam. In practice, in order to produce equivalent tissue ablation, this should translate to a higher laser power setting recommendation for the ProLase II compared with the Urolase and all other free-beam Nd:YAG delivery fibres used for coagulation prostatectomy, which have higher energy density beams.

In this quantitative study of Nd:YAG dosimetry in human prostates, it is found that a 40 W power setting and a minimum application time of 90 s produces maximal prostatic coagulation with the Urolase right-angle laser fibre (Figs 14.2 and 14.3). This confirms previous findings in the canine model.[9] By comparison, using the ProLase II side-firing laser fibre, it is found that a 60 W power setting and a minimum application time of 60 s produces maximal prostatic coagulation (Figs 14.2 and 14.3). Lower or higher power settings produce significantly less tissue effects with either device. Longer application times with either device produce relatively minimal increases in tissue effects, which are probably of no clinical significance.

The power dosimetry curve for the Urolase has a configuration and absolute amplitude almost identical to that produced with the ProLase II (Fig. 14.2), but the latter is shifted to the right on the horizontal axis by some 20 W (from 40 to 60 W). Similarly, the time dosimetry curve for the ProLase II mirrors that for the Urolase (Fig. 14.3), but is shifted to the left on the horizontal axis by some 30 s (from 90 to 60 s). This is consistent with the known variance in energy density of the Nd:YAG laser beam emitted by each fibre. With knowledge and application of this quantitative dosimetry data for each device, similar coagulative ablation of the prostate should be achievable with both. On the other hand, indiscriminate use of various laser settings, without attention to the individual delivery system beam characteristics, can potentially produce very different clinical outcomes. For example, use of the Urolase at a 60 W power setting or of the ProLase II at a 40 W power setting would significantly diminish tissue effects (Figs 14.2 and 14.3). The present data show that treatment parameters are not interchangeable beween fibres.

These quantitative dosimetry studies should now be extended to all other available laser delivery systems. Until this is done, there will be a continual problem with consistency and reproducibility of coagulation prostatectomy using different treatment devices.

References

1. Costello A J, Bowsher W G, Bolton D M et al. Laser ablation of the prostate in patients with benign prostatic hypertrophy. Br J Urol 1992; 69: 603–608
2. Cowles R S, Childs S, Dixon C et al. Prospective randomized study comparing transurethral resection of the prostate to visual laser ablation of the prostate. J Urol 1993; 149: 467A
3. Kabalin J N. Laser prostatectomy performed with a right angle firing neodymium:YAG laser fibre at 40 watts power setting. J Urol 1993; 150: 95–99
4. Norris J P, Norris D M, Lee R D, Rubenstein M A. Visual laser ablation of the prostate: clinical experience in 108 patients. J Urol 1993; 150: 1612–1614
5. Leach G E, Sirls L, Ganabathi K et al. Outpatient visual-assisted prostatectomy under local anaesthesia. Urology 1994; 43: 149–153
6. Costello A J, Shaffer B S, Crowe HR. Second-generation delivery systems for laser prostatic ablation. Urology 1994; 43: 262–266
7. Anson K M, Seenivasagam K, Watson G M. Visual laser ablation of prostate. Urology 1994; 43: 276
8. Shanberg A M, Lee I S, Tansey L A, Sawyer D E. Extensive neodymium:YAG photo-irradiaton of the prostate in men with obstructive prostatism. Urology 1994; 43: 467–471
9. Kabalin J N, Gill H S. Dosimetry studies utilizing the Urolase right angle firing neodymium:YAG laser fibre. Lasers Surg Med 1994; 14: 145–154
10. Kabalin J N, Gill H S. Urolase laser prostatectomy in patients on warfarin coagulation: a safe treatment alternative for bladder outlet obstruction. Urology 1993; 42: 738–740
11. Bolton D M, Costello A J. Management of benign prostatic hyperplasia by transurethral laser ablation in patients treated with warfarin anticoagulation. J Urol 1994; 151: 79–81

Dosimetry of a volume lesion in the canine prostate using Nd:YAG irradiation

15

A. P. Perlmutter   R. Muschter

Introduction

The use of neodymium:yttrium aluminium garnet (Nd:YAG) laser irradiation to perform a transurethral prostatectomy has become popular during the past few years owing to the development of several different types of laser delivery applicators that can be easily used through an endoscope. Many different treatment methods are currently evolving, and the various laser applicators include free-beam side-fire fibres, interstitial lightguides and contact vaporization tips.[1-3] The free-beam side-fire fibre can be used for tissue coagulation, vaporization and incision either alone or in combination.[4-8] Several feasibility studies and randomized clinical trials of transurethral resection of the prostate (TURP) have demonstrated the efficacy and safety of Nd:YAG laser prostatectomy.[9-12]

Laser irradiation causes thermal tissue destruction, and the different methods of laser application create different laser–tissue interactions. When free-beam side-fire fibres are used for coagulation, the goal of treatment is to accomplish heating deep into the prostate in order to coagulate the largest possible tissue volume. Optimal power and time parameters for maximum thermal penetration are only currently being elucidated.[13-18] The use of these fibres to create acute tissue vaporization requires that temperatures in excess of 100–300°C be reached at the tissue surface.[19] The authors have used the canine model to study the parameters involved in prostatic tissue destruction. Using a combination of video endoscopy, real time interstitial thermometry and acute pathology, the nature of the laser–tissue interaction during Nd:YAG irradiation can be defined.

Methods

All experiments were done using continuous-wave 1064 nm Nd:YAG lasers. The Urolase (Bard, Covington, GA, USA) and Ablaser (Microvasive, Watertown, MA, USA) in combination with Dornier 600 µm bare fibre were attached to the Fibertome 4060N laser (Dornier, Germering, Germany; provided at no cost by Dornier Medical Systems, Atlanta, GA, USA). New fibres, kindly provided at no cost by each manufacturer, were used for each experiment to avoid deterioration.

Temperature measurements were recorded in real time using copper–nickel–enamel thermocouples (Phillips, Hamburg, Germany). All data were directly computer recorded and graphed. The three thermocouples were mounted in a grid 4, 8 and 12 mm from a fixed laser fibre (Fig. 15.1). Direct Nd:YAG irradiation of the thermocouples in the grid under water at 40 W for 60 s resulted in a maximal temperature rise of 6°C at the

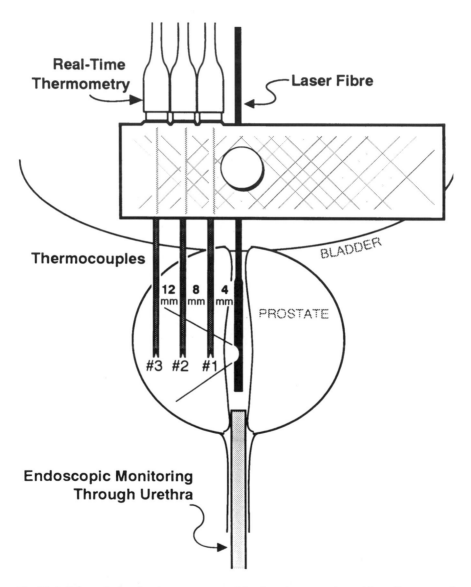

Fig. 15.1. Schematic showing the arrangement of the three thermocouples and laser fibre mounted in a device that holds all distances and orientations in the prostatic fossa constant. The thermocouples are 4 mm apart and, when the device is passed into the prostate during open surgery, the thermocouples are 3, 7 and 11 mm below the urothelial surface.

closest thermocouple and no temperature rise in the two distant thermocouples.

A series of 18 bred male beagles (12–24 kg) aged 2 years and older underwent open suprapubic cystotomy and perineal urethrostomy under general anaesthesia according to a protocol approved by the Institutional Animal Care and Use Committee. Care was taken to dissect the periprostatic space minimally in order to preserve vascular supply and thermal insulation. The free-beam side-fibre was fixed in the thermocouple grid and passed into the urethra while the thermocouple punctures were made in the lateral lobes (Fig. 15.1). The procedure was monitored by video endoscopy via a perineal urethrostomy with a 21 Fr cystoscope. Fibre placement in the urethra 1 mm from the tissue was estimated by noting the distance of the fibre from the urothelium compared with the known diameter of the fibre. Water at room temperature for irrigation was admitted through the cystoscope and was removed by suction from the bladder. Video monitoring allowed the observation of tissue change, 'popcorn' (see Results section) and carbonization, so that the time of these occurrences could be correlated with the temperature measurements. After the lasing procedure the dogs were killed, the prostates removed and 2–3 mm transverse sections prepared.

Results

Temperatures over 60–65°C cause protein denaturation and cell death.[20] Tissue blanching is seen endoscopically during this process, but the depth of coagulation is not known to the surgeon, who must empirically choose irradiation wattage and time treatment parameters. In order to assess the effect of increasing wattage (W), temperatures were measured at thermocouples 1, 2 and 3 during 30 s irradiations at 10, 20 and 40 W. Figure 15.2a shows that 10 W irradiation achieved only superficial coagulation by 30 s. Thermocouple 1 showed a virtually instantaneous temperature rise because of the thermal effect of direct laser light penetration into the tissue. The much smaller temperature rise at the next thermocouple, 4 mm deeper, confirmed that by 7 mm into the tissue there is little Nd:YAG light remaining. Video endoscopy during these temperature profiles revealed tissue blanching without popcorn or carbonization.

Irradiation at 20 W showed more rapid heating until popcorn without carbonization occurred, and then there was a subsequent temperature decrease to approximately 100°C (Fig. 15.2b). Popcorn, a frequent occurrence during continuous-wave laser irradiation, is due to the sudden formation of vapour below the intact urothelium. When the vapour pressure exceeds the internal tissue pressure, a crack forms to allow the vapour to be vented.[19] The thermometry during popcorn showed a temperature decrease due to mechanical heat dispersion and energy consumption during the phase change; however, deep tissue reheating was re-established.

(a)

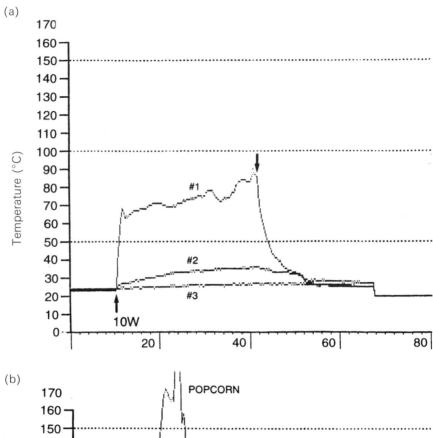

(b)

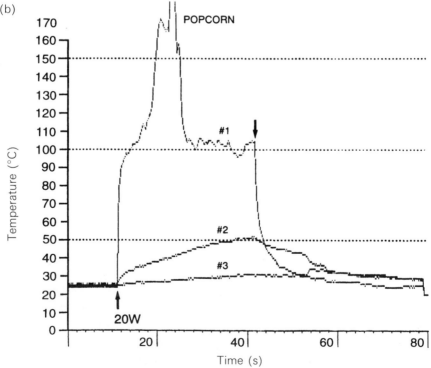

(c)

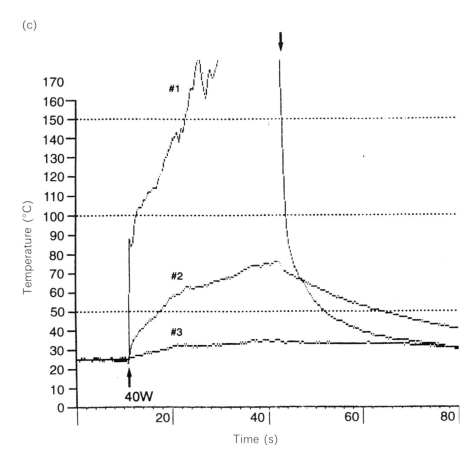

Fig. 15.2. (a and b opposite) Time–temperature profiles in the canine model. The beginning and end of lasing is denoted by the heavy arrows. Irradiation for 30 s with the Ablaser catheter was at (a) 10 W, (b) 20 W and (c) 40 W.

Figure 15.2c shows that 40 W irradiation created even higher superficial temperatures without carbonization, and coagulation temperature was exceeded at the middle thermocouple by 30 s. In spite of excellent heating by thermal conduction to the middle thermocouple, the deepest thermocouple did not demonstrate a significant temperature rise. The probable explanation is that in this living, perfused canine model, tissue blood flow dissipates thermal energy in the peripheral prostate, and a balance is reached between the influx of heat and efferent cooling.

In order to investigate the ability of longer irradiation times to heat deeper into the prostate, 20 and 40 W irradiations were studied for 3 min. Figure 15.3a shows that longer irradiation times allowed temperatures to increase very slowly at the deepest thermocouple; however, coagulation temperatures were not achieved. The popcorn event caused a temperature fall at thermocouple 1, and temperature increased at thermocouple 2

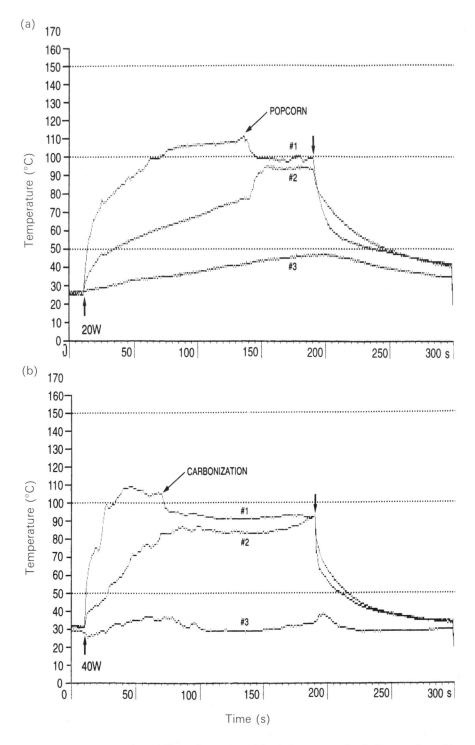

Fig. 15.3. Time–temperature profiles in the canine model. The beginning and end of lasing is denoted by the heavy arrows. Irradiation for 3 min with the Urolase catheter was at (a) 20 W and (b) 40 W.

because the tissue explosion removed some of the intervening prostate tissue. The effect of carbonization can be seen in Fig. 15.3b. Endoscopy revealed a small amount of tissue vaporization with carbonization. The effect of carbonization was seen at thermocouple 3 as a decrease in temperature. Despite continued irradiation, thermocouple 2 did not undergo any increase in temperature, despite irradiation for a total of 3 min.

In order to achieve tissue vaporization, higher temperatures must be reached. This process is intimately linked to tissue carbonization, which occurs on the tissue surface and is due to the pyrolysis and combustion of organic molecules at temperatures in the range of 100–300°C.[19,20] When this dark material forms on the surface, there is intense superficial absorption of the laser energy and thus rapid heating to temperatures that cause tissue vaporization. Figure 15.4 shows the acute gross pathology after vaporization. The hyperaemic rim, which approximates to the depth of coagulation, can be seen to extend only 2–3 mm beyond the vaporized cavity. Thus, when high laser powers and high energy density were used to vaporize tissue, concomitant deeper coagulation was not achieved.

Discussion

Laser prostatectomy is a technique in evolution. Some approaches aim to coagulate the maximum volume of prostate tissue, whereas others use vaporization alone or in combination with coagulation. Thus, depending on the surgical goal, different types of laser–tissue interaction are desirable. The results reported here allow insight into the effect of wattage, popcorn

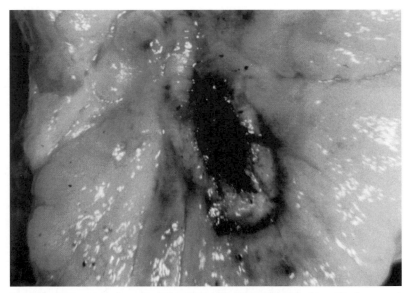

Fig. 15.4. Acute gross pathology of a lesion vaporized with the Urolase fibre. The hyperaemic rim extends only 2–3 mm beyond the cavity.

and vaporization on the formation of a volume lesion in the canine prostate.

The canine prostate is a commonly used model system for laser experimentation because it is difficult to perform carefully measured fixed-distance lasing in humans, with hand-held cystoscopes. However, the canine prostate is more glandular and completes the cycle of Nd:YAG-induced necrosis, tissue sloughing and re-epithelialization in less time than its human counterpart.[21,22] In addition, the measured coagulation lesion to the hyperaemic rim may not correlate to the final lesion size. Although not a perfect model, the principles of heat transfer and tissue destruction are similar. There is probably not an exact correlation of laser–tissue interaction at a given wattage between the human and canine systems, but the trends and observations should hold true.

Interstitial thermometry allows several clinical recommendations for undertaking a free-beam side-fire coagulation prostatectomy. The data clearly shows that higher temperature profiles penetrate deeper as wattage is increased from 10 to 40 W. This occurs as long as the only visualized tissue change is blanching with some tissue contraction. The authors found that the depth of the lesion was not linearly proportional to irradiation time: there was an initial, rapid temperature rise leading to coagulation to a moderate depth, followed by slower depth expansion. It is likely that the first phase is the effect of direct irradiation and the second phase is heat conduction from the surface lesion. Clinically, therefore, the maximum depth of penetration is obtained by the highest wattage that does not carbonize or vaporize.

The popcorn event in the canine prostate was associated with a transient decrease in superficial temperatures; however, it was not associated with the loss in the ability to heat deep into the gland. Carbonization limited the temperature rise deep in the prostate, and thus should be avoided in any technique that uses coagulation as the primary mode of tissue destruction. The depth of tissue heating is the most important factor limiting the total volume of tissue that can be coagulated. The surgeon who desires coagulation should react to the formation of carbon by decreasing lasing power or by slightly increasing the distance between the tissue and laser fibre in order to reduce the effective laser power density. However, carbonization is an instrumental step in the formation of a vaporized lesion, and thus should not be avoided during such techniques. Gross pathology showed that there was little coagulation beyond 3 mm of a vaporized carbonized cavity.

Laser prostatectomy is dynamic surgery, not a cookbook. The surgeon can react to observed laser–tissue interactions during the procedure and modify the lasing protocol in order to obtain the results desired.

Acknowledgements

Research was supported by the Department of Urology and the James Buchanan Brady Foundation, New York Hospital–Cornell Medical Center.

References

1. Costello A J, Bowsher W G, Bolton D M et al. Laser ablation of the prostate in patients with benign prostatic hypertrophy. Br J Urol 1992; 69: 603–608
2. Muschter R. Lasers and benign prostatic hyperplasia—experimental and clinical results to compare different application systems. J Urol 1994; 151: 230A
3. Gomella LG, Lofti M A. Contact laser vaporization of the prostate for benign prostatic hypertrophy. SPIE Proc 1994; 2129: 99–105
4. Kabalin J N. Laser prostatectomy performed with a right angle firing neodymium:YAG laser fibre at 40 watts power setting. J Urol 1993; 150: 95–99
5. Childs S J. Laser-assisted transurethral resection of the prostate. Baltimore: Williams & Wilkins, 1993
6. McCullough D L, Roth R A, Babayan R K et al. Transurethral ultrasound-guided laser-induced prostatectomy: National Human Cooperative Study results. J Urol 1993; 150: 1607–1611
7. Daughtry J D, Rodan B A. A comparison of contact tip mode and lateral firing free beam mode. J Clin Laser Med Surg 1993; 11: 21–27
8. Narayan P, Fournier G, Indudhara R et al. Transurethral evaporation of prostate (TUEP) with Nd:YAG laser using a contact free beam technique: results in 61 patients with benign prostatic hyperplasia. Urology 1994; 43: 813–820
9. Costello A J, Crowe H R. A single institution experience of reflecting laser prostatectomy over 4 years. J Urol 1994; 151: 229A
10. Dixon C. Right-angle free beam lasers for the treatment of benign prostatic hyperplasia. Semin Urol 1994; 12: 165–169
11. Leach G E, Dmochowski R, Ganabathi K et al. Visual laser assisted prostatectomy (VLAP) using Urolase right angle fiber: multicenter 60 watt protocol. J Urol 1994; 151: 228A
12. Dixon C, Marchi G, Theune C et al. A prospective, double-blind, randomized study comparing the safety, efficacy, and cost of laser ablation of the prostate and transurethral prostatectomy for the treatment of BPH. J Urol 1994; 151: 229A
13. Cammack J T, Motamedi M, Torres J H et al. Endoscopic Nd:YAG laser coagulation of the prostate: comparison of low power versus high power. J Urol 1993; 149: 215A
14. Anvari B, Motamedi M, Torres J et al. Optical properties of native and coagulated canine prostate. Lasers Surg Med 1993; (suppl): 64
15. Kabalin J N, Gill H S. Dosimetry studies utilizing the Urolase right angle firing neodymium:YAG laser fiber. Lasers Surg Med 1994; 14: 145–154
16. Shanberg A M, Lee I S, Tansey L A et al. Depth of penetration of the neodymium:yttrium–aluminum–garnet laser in the human prostate at various dosimetry. Urology 1994; 43: 809–812
17. Perlmutter A P, Muschter R. The optimization of laser prostatectomy part I: free beam side fire coagulation. Urology 1994; 44: 847–855
18. Muschter R, Perlmutter A P. The optimization of laser prostatectomy part II: other lasing techniques. Urology 1994; 44: 856–861
19. Verdaasdonk R M, Borst C, Van Gemert M J C. Explosive onset of continuous wave laser tissue ablation. Phys Med Biol 1990; 35: 1129–1144
20. Stein B S. Laser physics and tissue interaction. In: Smith J A, Stein B S, Benson R C (eds) Lasers in urologic surgery. Chicago: Year Book Medical, 1989: 1–22
21. Johnson D E, Price R E, Cromeens D M. Pathologic changes occurring in the prostate following transurethral laser prostatectomy. Lasers Surg Med 1992; 12: 254–263
22. Marks L. Serial endoscopy following visual laser ablation of prostate (VLAP). Urology 1993; 42: 66–71

Clinical outcome of symptomatic BPH patients treated by TULIP or TURP: a prospective and randomized study

16

H. Schulze   W. Martin   T. Senge

Introduction

Benign prostatic hyperplasia (BPH) can be detected in 68% of men over 50 years old.[1] Evidence of BPH as determined by transrectal ultrasound and/or obstructive voiding symptoms exists in 43% of all men between 60 and 69 years old.[2] During the last decades, transurethral resection of the prostate (TURP) has become the most frequently used mode of surgical treatment for bladder outlet obstruction due to BPH.

Many technical improvements have reduced the postoperative mortality rate following TURP to less than 1%. However, several studies have shown that morbidity following TURP has remained stable at about 20% for the last 30 years.[3–8] Thus, despite the high degree of efficacy of TURP, the concomitant intra- and postoperative morbidity have encouraged urologists to consider alternative treatment forms that would ideally be as effective as TURP but would have fewer side effects.

In 1986, Kandel and associates reported for the first time the use of the neodymium:yttrium aluminium garnet (Nd:YAG) laser specifically to treat BPH in dogs.[9] Four years later Roth, Aretz and Lage presented a more sophisticated device to relieve bladder outlet obstruction due to enlargement of the prostate; this device is known as TULIP, an acronym for transurethral ultrasound-guided laser-induced prostatectomy.[10] The TULIP system combines a real time ultrasound transducer and a Nd:YAG laser delivery system within a 20 Fr urethral probe. Also in 1990, the first TULIP procedures in men with symptomatic obstructive BPH were performed in the United States and shortly thereafter also in Europe.[11] Several investigators have now reported their first experiences with this new device.[12–17] It has become clear that, in the majority of patients, subjective and/or objective symptoms have improved following TULIP, and that this mode of treatment may have advantages as well as disadvantages compared with TURP, which is considered the gold standard treatment modality in BPH. Meanwhile, clinical results have been published demonstrating the durability of TULIP outcome at a 2 year

161

follow-up.[18] However, for direct comparison of TULIP and TURP prospective, randomized studies are required according to guidelines suggested by the American Urological Association (AUA).[19]

The TULIP device

The TULIP system (Intra-Sonix, Inc., Burlington, MA, USA) represents the combination of a real time ultrasound transducer and a Nd:YAG laser delivery system within a 20 Fr transurethral probe. The 7.5 MHz ultrasound transducer produces a 90 degree sector image of the prostate. The laser prism reflects the laser beam in a 90 degree angle from the probe towards the tissue at the centre of the ultrasound sector.

During use, the distal end of the transurethral probe is covered by a special sterile disposable sleeve, at the end of which is a balloon (available in either 36 or 48 Fr when inflated). The proximal part of the probe fits into a control handle that enables the operator to move the laser aperture and transducer in both axial and radial directions.

Before and after TULIP a cystoscopy is performed. The probe, with the sleeve in place, is introduced into the prostatic urethra like a resectoscope and is stabilized by filling the sleeve with sterile water pressurized to two atmospheres (≈ 202 kPa). This creates a smooth tissue surface and a distance between the laser aperture and the tissue, thus ensuring an optimal ultrasound image and a set, controlled and constant laser beam diameter. The probe can be coupled to most of the existing continuous-wave Nd:YAG lasers.

The prostatic tissue is heated by the laser irradiation. A laser power setting of 30–40 W is chosen to induce coagulation necrosis. The procedure is virtually bloodless and the necrotic tissue is excreted in the urine for approximately 4–6 weeks after the procedure. However, the TULIP procedure does not produce an acute improvement of micturition: in most cases, micturition is impaired in the early postoperative phase, probably owing to oedema of the prostatic tissue. For this reason a suprapubic catheter is inserted during the procedure. In most cases this catheter can be removed at the time of the first postoperative assessment after 3 weeks. Dexamethasone (3×8 mg on the day of operation) and anti-inflammatory drugs (e.g. diclofenac 2×50 mg p.o./day for 2–3 weeks) are administered.

Patients and methods

A total of 41 patients admitted to the authors' department because of obstructive and symptomatic BPH were included in a prospective and randomized study to compare the efficacy and side effects of TULIP (n=20) versus TURP (n=21). Inclusion and exclusion criteria are shown in Table 16.1.

Inclusion criteria*	Exclusion criteria
• Symptomatic, obstructive BPH (DRE and TRUS not suspicious, PSA < 10 ng/ml or benign prostatic biopsy)	• Patient age > 75 years
	• Prostate volume < 25 cm^3 or > 75 cm^3
	• Neurogenic micturition disorder
	• Bladder stone
• Peak urine flow < 15 ml/s	• Bladder cancer
• Residual urine > 30 ml	• Previous prostatic or urethral surgery
• Modified Boyarsky symptom score > 15/36	• Patient refusal of randomization procedure

Table 16.1. Inclusion and exclusion criteria for patients in a prospective and randomized study of the efficacy and side effects of transurethral ultrasound-guided laser-induced prostatectomy (TULIP) and of transurethral resection of the prostate (TURP)

*BPH, benign prostatic hyperplasia; DRE, digital rectal examination; TRUS, transrectal ultrasound; PSA, prostate-specific antigen.

Preoperative data showed an equal distribution between the two groups (patient age 64.5 vs 65.9 years; prostate volume 48.4 vs 50.1 cm^3; urinary peak flow 3.2 vs 2.4 ml/s; residual urine volume: 371 vs 347 ml; symptom score 19.0 vs 17.7, in the TULIP and TURP groups, respectively), with 13 patients being in urinary retention prior to treatment in each group. All procedures were performed under peridural anaesthesia.

Intra- and postoperative data are shown in Table 16.2. On average, laser treatment took 20 min less than TURP. The estimated blood loss was 51 ml during TULIP and 515 ml during TURP. The haemoglobin value was virtually the same before and after operation in the TULIP group (from 14.4 to 14.5 g/l), whereas after TURP there was a fall of 2 g/l on average (from 14.5 to 12.4 g/l). However, in no case in either group was a blood transfusion necessary. Length of hospital stay favoured TULIP-treated patients (2.7 vs 6.8 days). On the other hand, the suprapubic catheter, which was placed in every patient before operation, was removed after TURP at the time of discharge (6.7 days) whereas, because of initially inadequate micturition, after TULIP it was left in place for nearly 5 weeks (34.1 days). At the first follow-up visit after 3 weeks, 30% of the TULIP patients (6/20) still had urinary retention.

During further follow-up, retrograde ejaculation in sexually active men was reported by 31% of the TULIP-treated patients (4/13) and by 50% of the TURP-treated patients (4/8).

Results

Results obtained during the first year after the procedure in both treatment groups regarding symptom score and urinary peak flow are shown in Figs 16.1 and 16.2. After 3 months, residual urine volume decreased to approximately 50 and 25 ml in the TULIP and TURP groups, respectively, and remained

| Data | Treatment* | |
	TULIP	TURP
Procedural time (min)	32 (12–55)	52 (30–95)
Irrigation vol (l)	1.4 (1–2.5)	22 (6–32)
Laser passes (no.)	9 (8–12)	—
Laser energy (J)	14 500 (11 800–22 500)	—
Resected volume (cm³)	—	36.2 (12–60)
Blood loss (ml)	51 (10–150)	515 (150–1200)
Haemoglobin (g/l)		
Preop	14.4	14.5
Postop	14.5	12.4
Hospital stay (days)	2.7 (1–7)	6.8 (2–20)
Suprapubic catheter (days)	34.1 (9–90)	6.7 (2–19)
Urine retention 3 weeks postop [percentage of patients]	30 [6/20]	0
Retrograde ejaculation [percentage of patients]	31 [4/13]	50 [4/8]

Table 16.2. Intraoperative and postoperative data of 41 patients undergoing TULIP (n=20) or TURP (n=21) for BPH

*Ranges in parentheses.

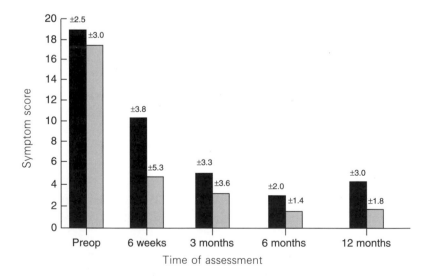

Fig. 16.1. Symptom score (assessed by modified Boyarsky score) within the first postoperative year in patients undergoing either transurethral ultrasound-guided laser-induced prostatectomy (TULIP; ■) or transurethral resection of the prostate (TURP; ■). Values above columns are ±SD.

164

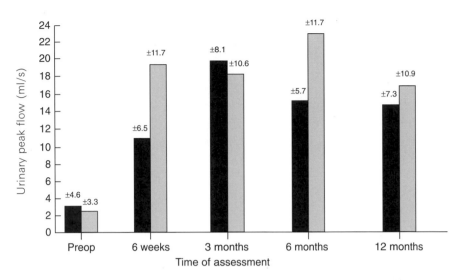

Fig. 16.2. Mean urinary peak flow within the first postoperative year in patients undergoing either TULIP; ■ or TURP; ▨). Values above columns are ±SD.

stable during further follow-up. Overall (a) there is a substantial improvement of each parameter in both groups, (b) the improvement in each parameter is even more pronounced in the TURP group than in the TULIP group, and (c) for the laser-treated patients it takes considerably longer to achieve results that are nearly comparable to the improvements seen after TURP (approximately 3 months).

However, if a reduction of more than 50% in total symptom score after 6 months is taken as an indication of successful treatment, the rate of successfully treated patients is the same in both groups [for TULIP, 18/18 patients (100%), score falling from 19.1 to 3.0; for TURP, 17/18 patients (94%), score falling from 17.6 to 1.8]. The same is true with respect to urinary peak flow if a peak flow of more than 15 ml/s is required [for TULIP, 12/17 patients (71%), peak flow increasing from 4.2 to 18.5 ml/s; for TURP, 12/17 patients (71%), peak flow increasing from 3.4 to 27.9 ml/s]. If both requirements (symptom score reduction >50% plus urinary peak flow >15 ml/s) are combined, again the rate of thus-defined successfully treated patients is the same—71% (12/17 patients) in both treatment groups.

Prostate volume reduction

In 13 and 12 patients, respectively, prostate volume was determined before and 6 months after the procedure using transrectal ultrasound. The decrease in prostate volume after TURP was double that after TULIP [TULIP, from 49.5 to 35.3 cm^3 (-28.7%); TURP, from 54.6 to 21.1 cm^3 (-61.4%)].

Complications

As already mentioned, no blood transfusion was necessary in either group. Moreover, no post-transurethral resection syndrome was observed in any patient in this study.

In the TULIP group there was one case of epididymitis and one of second-degree stress incontinence. In one patient a TURP was performed 18 months after the TULIP procedure. In addition, one patient died 22 days after the procedure from myocardial infarction; there was no evidence that this was related to TULIP.

In the TURP group, in two cases a second TURP was performed 1 week after the first procedure, because of inadequate micturition; in another case, clot retention occurred 3 weeks after the procedure and in two cases urethral strictures required internal urethrotomy 4 and 6 months after the TURP, respectively.

Discussion

Laser therapy for treatment of bladder outlet obstruction due to BPH has gained increasing attention in the last few years. For decades transrectal resection of the prostate was considered the 'gold standard', but careful analysis revealed that rates of side effects and complications after TURP were higher than most urologists would have thought. As different forms of laser therapy, nearly all using the Nd:YAG laser for removal of BPH tissue, have become available the question arises whether this new form of treatment will bring about clinical results comparable to those with TURP, at the same time substantially reducing the morbidity of the procedure. Meanwhile, the results of many phase II studies have been reported and published, demonstrating that laser treatment is capable of relieving bladder outlet obstruction. However, data of prospective and randomized studies comparing laser therapy with TURP are still rare.

The results of the randomized, prospective study described here reveals advantages as well as disadvantages of TULIP in comparison to TURP. In favour of TULIP are length of hospital stay (TULIP may even be performed on an outpatient basis), intraoperative blood loss and rate of retrograde ejaculation. On the other hand, delayed onset of success, long duration of catherization required (often combined with irritative symptoms during the early postoperative phase) and less prostate volume reduction (compared with TURP) are (or may be) disadvantages.

In comparison with symptoms before treatment, TULIP and TURP both demonstrated substantial improvements in subjective as well as in objective symptoms. However, those improvements seen were even more pronounced after TURP. Success rates, as defined in this study (symptom score reduction more than 50% and peak urinary flow more than 15 ml/s after 6 months), on the other hand, were the same after TULIP and after TURP treatment.

With regard to complications, there is increasing evidence that every effective mode of treatment of obstructive BPH will also cause some side effects and morbidity. This is also true of all types of laser treatment currently under clinical investigation. In addition, it has to be emphasized that all published complication rates regarding TURP are based on procedures performed in the 1980s or earlier. Technical improvements have reduced TURP complications, as demonstrated in this study of TULIP vs TURP, leading to a similar rate of complications after laser treatment and transurethral resection.

In addition, it must be borne in mind that, when using TULIP (and the same is true for every other laser or thermotherapy procedure), no tissue is obtained for histological evaluation. Despite the use of protein-specific antigen (PSA) determination and monitoring with transrectal ultrasound (TRUS), the rate of incidental prostate cancer in the authors' department following TURP is about 6%. It is not known whether those missed incidental prostate cancers may become clinically important in the future, but young patients, in particular, should be followed up very carefully after TULIP treatment, or after any other form of laser treatment in which no tissue is obtained for histological evaluation.

Finally, it should be emphasized that the long-term effect of any form of laser treatment is still unknown; this information is necessary before any final conclusions can be drawn regarding the efficacy and cost effectiveness of such treatments.

In conclusion, as demonstrated in phase II studies and now in this randomized study, TULIP gives rise to a significant improvement in symptoms of urine flow obstruction. In comparison with symptoms before treatment, improvements (in urinary peak flow, residual urine volume and symptom score) obtained by TURP are (a) even more pronounced and (b) occur nearly immediately after the procedure, whereas after laser treatment the patient must wait for 6 weeks to 3 months before noting improvement. In favour of TULIP are reduced blood loss, hospitalization and rate of postoperative sexual dysfunction. The rates of intra- and postoperative complications, however, are very similar in both groups, although this is difficult to evaluate because of the small number of patients included in this study.

References

1. Berry S J, Coffey, D S, Walsh P C, Ewing L L. The development of human benign prostatic hyperplasia with age. J Urol 1984; 132: 474–479
2. Garraway W M, Collins G N, Lee R J. High prevalence of benign prostatic hypertrophy in the community. Lancet 1991; 338: 469–471
3. Holtgrewe H L, Valk W L. Factors influencing the mortality and morbidity of transurethral prostatectomy: a study of 2,015 cases. J Urol 1962; 87: 450–459
4. Melchior J, Valk W L, Foret J D, Mebust W K. Transurethral prostatectomy: computerized analysis of 2,223 consecutive cases. J Urol 1974; 112: 634–642

5. Mebust W K, Holtgrewe H L, Cockett A T K et al. Transurethral prostatectomy: immediate and postoperative complications. A cooperative study of 13 participating institutions evaluating 3,885 patients. J Urol 1989; 141: 243–247

6. Holtgrewe H L, Mebust W K, Dowd J B et al. Transurethral prostatectomy: practice aspects of the dominant operation in American urology. J Urol 1989; 141: 248–253

7. Pientka L, Van Loghem J, Hahn E, Keil U. Häufigkeit und Komplikationen der Prostataadenomchirurgie bei Patienten mit benigner Prostatahyperplasie. Urologe [B] 1991; 31: 211–216

8. Doll H A, Black N A, McPherson K et al. Mortality, morbidity and complications following transurethral resection of the prostate for benign prostatic hypertrophy. J Urol 1992; 147: 1566–1573

9. Kandel L B, Harrison L H, McCullough D L et al. Transurethral laser prostatectomy: creation of a technique for using the neodymium:yttrium aluminum garnet (YAG) laser in the canine model. J Urol 1986; 135: 110A

10. Roth R A, Aretz H T. Transurethral ultrasound-guided laser-induced prostatectomy (TULIP procedure): a canine prostate feasibility study. J Urol 1991; 146: 1128–1135

11. Schulze H. TULIP—transurethral ultrasound-guided laser-induced prostatectomy. World J Urol 1995; in press

12. McCullough D L, Roth R A, Babayan R K et al. Transurethral ultrasound-guided laser-induced prostatectomy: national human cooperative study results. J Urol 1993; 150: 1607–1611

13. Homma Y, Takahashi S, Minowada S, Aso Y. Treating benign prostatic hyperplasia with transurethral ultrasound-guided laser induced prostatectomy (TULIP). Urol Surg Tokyo 1993; 6: 97–106

14. Schulze H, Martin W, Engelmann U, Senge T. TULIP—transurethrale ultraschallgeführte laserinduzierte Prostatektomie: eine Alternative zur TURP? Urologe [A] 1993; 32: 225–231

15. De la Rosette J J M C H, Froeling F M J A, Alivizatos G, Debruyne F M J. Laser ablation of the prostate: experience with an ultrasound guided technique and a procedure under direct vision. Eur Urol 1994; 25: 19–24

16. Puppo P, Perachino M, Ricciotti G, Scannapieco G. Transurethral ultrasound-guided laser-induced prostatectomy. Eur Urol 1984; 25: 220–225

17. Schulze H, Martin W, Hoch P et al. Transurethral ultrasound-guided laser-induced prostatectomy: clinical outcome and data analyses. Urology 1995; in press

18. Babayan R K, Roth R A, McCullough D L et al. TULIP—two year results. J Urol 1994; 151: 228A

19. Holtgrewe H L. Guidance for clinical investigations of devices used for the treatment of benign prostatic hyperplasia. J Urol 1993; 150: 1588–1590

One year follow-up of 80 patients undergoing visual laser ablation of the prostate

17

R. S. Cowles III

Introduction

Benign prostatic hyperplasia (BPH) resulting in bladder outlet obstruction is one of the most significant problems affecting men today. In the United States almost one-third of all men will undergo prostatectomy by the eighth decade of life. Over 400 000 transurethral prostatectomies are performed per year.[1]

The unquestioned efficacy of transurethral resection of the prostate (TURP) has made it the 'gold standard' for the treatment of bladder outlet obstruction secondary to BPH over the past 60 years worldwide. However, TURP does have a significant complication rate. The American Urological Association (AUA) Cooperative Study[2] has reported an 18% immediate postoperative morbidity rate. Although pre- and postoperative medical therapy, together with anaesthesia, has improved significantly, this complication rate has remained relatively constant over the past 30 years.[3]

For this reason, investigators began to look for alternative means of therapy to treat bladder outlet obstruction. Until recently, technology was not available to introduce laser energy into the prostate adequately. Johnson et al[4] performed canine studies using a right-angle firing delivery system. This allowed neodymium:yttrium aluminium garnet (Nd:YAG) laser energy to penetrate the prostate, resulting in coagulative necrosis of the prostatic tissue, which over the course of time was noted to slough, creating a large spherical ectatic cavity in the prostate.[4]

An initial multicentre trial utilized a prospective randomized trial comparing TURP with visual laser ablation of the prostate (VLAP). Prostates were treated with 40 W for 30 s in the 12 and 6 o'clock positions and 40 W for 60 s in the 3 and 9 o'clock positions. The results of this study were presented at the 1993 AUA annual convention. This study demonstrated the safety and efficacy of this procedure compared with TURP.[5]

Patients and methods

Eighty patients were selected who met conventional criteria indicating a need for surgical intervention to treat bladder outlet obstruction secondary to BPH. Patients underwent baseline or preoperative evaluation using the

AUA-6 symptom score questionnaire,[6] peak voiding flow rate and post-voiding residual urine determinations.

Patients with suspected BPH based on an abnormal rectal examination or elevation of prostate-specific antigen (PSA >4.0) first underwent transrectal ultrasonography and prostate biopsy, and were excluded if found to have adenocarcinoma of the prostate. Patients deemed unfit for either regional or general anaesthesia were excluded from this study.

Operative time was recorded as beginning when the lasing was started and concluding upon placement of a Foley catheter.

The Urolase® 90 degree angle reflecting fibre was used in all patients. This fibre is a 600 μm quartz fibre with a gold-plate reflecting tip; the angle of reflection is 90 degrees. All cases were performed under videoscopy as opposed to direct vision. Patients received either general or regional anaesthesia.

The average operative time was 22 min. One new laser fibre was used per procedure, and no additional laser fibre was required for any patient. Average fibre degradation, as measured on the power meter, was 13%.

Technique

Although all urologists are familiar with the use of the cystoscope in the prostatic fossa, this is a new procedure and thus employs different manoeuvres using the cystoscope and laser fibre in order to treat the prostate adequately. Because of this new and different technique, a detailed description is given here to aid in the understanding of this surgical experience.

Once the laser and fibre have been confirmed to be fully operational, the patient is then anaesthetized and placed in the dorsal lithotomy position. Water is used as irrigant in the VLAP procedure as there is no reabsorption of irrigating fluid. A pressure cuff is placed about the irrigation solution to improve the flow of irrigant in large prostates or difficult procedures. The decision to inflate the pressure cuff is based soley on the ease of irrigation of the laser fibre during the procedure. Care should be taken not to overinflate the bladder with irrigant, especially in compromised or non-compliant bladders, to prevent rupture.

A 21 Fr cystoscope with a 30 degree lens is used as the 7.5 Fr fibre fits easily through this size cystoscope. Although larger scopes can be used, they tend to be more traumatic to the urethra, and without special stabilizing devices in the cystoscope the laser fibre tends to have more mobility and less control in larger rather than smaller cystoscopes.

The use of video as opposed to direct vision is important in this procedure, for several reasons. The use of videoscopy allows the urological surgeon to wear the appropriate eye protective glasses without hindering his view through the cystoscope. Second, during this procedure the cystoscope is held in various positions in the prostatic fossa to which the urologist may not be accustomed and this may make direct vision difficult secondary to positioning of the cystoscope. If the surgeon is unaccustomed to videoscopy it is recommended that this technique and VLAP should be learned independently.

Gentle cystoscopy is extremely important in this procedure, as bleeding not only can damage the laser fibre but also may cause some decrease in absorption of laser energy. The inspection of the bladder and urethra before beginning the laser treatment should be done with care and as atraumatically as possible.

The Nd:YAG laser is set at 60 W and each lasing quadrant is lased for 60 s. A stopwatch is used to calculate the exact time of laser energy delivery. The lasing quadrants are 2, 4, 8 and 10 o'clock. If the prostate is envisaged as the face of a clock, the verumontanum is in the 6 o'clock position. Once lasing has begun, it is important to try to complete 60 s lasing without stopping the procedure. Short pauses are acceptable; however, discontinuing lasing prior to completion of the 60 s burn may result in decreased heat penetration and of the subsequent coagulative necrotic effect.

Before lasing is started, a complete operative plan should be formulated regarding how many lasing quadrants will be required to treat the prostate. Prostates less than 3 cm in length from bladder neck to verumontanum are lased in one 'round-the-clock' fashion, i.e. at 2, 4, 8 and 10 o'clock in a mid-gland position (halfway between the bladder neck and verumontanum lasings (see Fig. 17.1). Larger prostates can be lased using two or three 'round-the-clock' lasings. Once again, understanding the physics and dosimetry of this technique is crucial to the correct performance of VLAP.

Because of the three-dimensional nature of the coagulative necrotic effect caused by the laser energy it is crucial not to lase the prostate distal to the verumontanum, to avoid possible damage to, or obliteration of, the

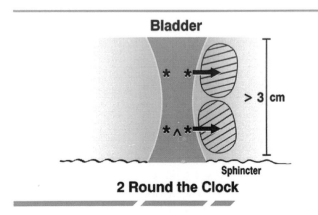

Fig. 17.1. Prostate, with two 'round-the-clock' lasings.

external sphincter. If, as in many cases, there is doubt about the need for one or two 'round-the-clock' lasings based on prostatic size, twice rather than once is recommended, on the basis that any overlap of coagulative necrotic effect does not increase the depth of penetration but merely causes coagulative necrosis in an area that has already been treated. Thus, increasing the number of lasing quadrants does not, in fact, increase the risk of damage outside the prostatic capsule but merely requires more time and may cause further degradation of the laser fibre.

Median lobes and high bladder necks are easily treated. A median bar can be treated with 60 W for 60 s in the 6 o'clock position. Small median lobes are treated safely in the 6 o'clock position at 60 W for 60 s. A larger median lobe can be treated in the 5 and 7 o'clock positions, 60 W for 60 s in each lasing position. Median lobes that are even larger can be treated in the 5, 6 and 7 o'clock positions, and extremely large median lobes can subsequently be treated in a T-fashion, 60 W for 60 s in each lasing position.

Four concepts are important to remember before beginning to lase in each particular quadrant. First, the fibre itself should be in the correct 2, 4, 8 or 10 o'clock position. Second, as fibres are angled delivery systems, the rotation of the fibre in its relationship to the prostate laser quadrant is critical; the holding device on the fibre is very helpful in maintaining tactile control. Third, the distance of the fibre from the end of the cystoscope is extremely important: if the fibre is too close to the cystoscope, either the telescope or the cystoscope can be damaged from the heat energy of the laser; if the fibre is too far from the end of the cystoscope, vision is impaired, as is irrigation of the laser fibre. The urologist should, therefore, be able to see the entire tip of the laser fibre being used, so that it can be irrigated appropriately and its burial in tissue (which can be detrimental to the life of the fibre) can be avoided. Fourth, the distance of the fibre tip from the prostate is important. The tip should never adhere to the prostatic tissue, otherwise rapid degradation of the fibre can ensue secondary to decreased irrigation of the tip. In addition, such adherence creates both tissue char and protein denaturation, resulting in decreased depth of penetration of the laser energy; the tip should be held as close as possible to the prostatic tissue without adherence. In order to prevent adherence, cystoscopic deflection, as described below, including use of the pressure cuff on the irrigating solution while lasing, is crucial to the survival of the laser tip. To confirm the 'freedom' of the fibre, a 'flick of the wrist' (1–2 mm) rapid movement of the fibre can be very helpful.

In VLAP, the cystoscope can be used as a tool to place the laser fibre in the appropriate position, as well as to manipulate the prostate to prevent damage to the laser fibre. The positioning and various aspects of placement of the laser fibre in the prostatic fossa have been described above. The use of 'cystoscopic deflection' of the prostate is critical to achieve proper placement of the laser fibre in certain cases. This cystoscopic deflection can be described as either 'fulcrum' deflection or 'in parallel' deflection. The fulcrum deflection of the cystoscope is one commonly employed by urologists in order to view the dome of the bladder or the base of the bladder. This essentially is an up-and-down, or 12 and 6 o'clock, movement of the cystoscope. Clearly, when lasing in the 2 and 10 o'clock positions, the cystoscope is in the 'fulcrum up' position and, conversely, 'fulcrum down' to lase in the 4 and 8 o'clock positions. In smaller prostates this type of deflection may be all that is necessary in order to achieve proper placement of the laser fibre. However, in lasing larger prostates the lateral lobes are commonly found to abut each other in the midline. This makes it difficult to pass the laser fibre past the beak of the cystoscope so that adequate vision of the entire laser tip is obtained without 'burying' the fibre tip in the prostatic tissue. It is in precisely this circumstance where 'in parallel' deflection of the cystoscope is crucial. By grasping the cystoscope and deflecting the entire cystoscope in parallel with the plane of the urethra and prostate, the contralateral obstructing lobe can be pushed aside to an extent sufficient to allow adequate vision, irrigation and placement of the laser fibre so that it is not enveloped by the lateral lobes. Several millimetres of movement from the lateral lobe should not be expected; however, 1–2 mm is suffice to achieve proper placement of the laser tip. Thus if, for example, the 2 o'clock position is to be lased, then the operator would not only 'fulcrum up' the cystoscope but would also 'in parallel' deflect the right lateral lobe using the cystoscope, exposing the surface of the left lateral lobe to achieve proper placement of the laser fibre (Fig. 17.2).

This also illustrates another important difference in VLAP and TURP with respect to cystoscope placement. In performing TURP, the

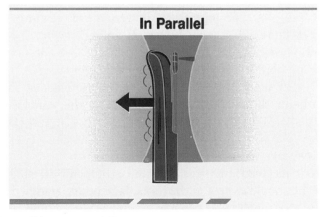

Fig. 17.2. In parallel cystoscopic deflection.

resectoscope is rotated circumferentially inside the prostatic fossa. However, during VLAP the cystoscope should be maintained in the up-and-down (or 12 to 6 o'clock) position. The only rotation that is necessary is that of the laser fibre; there is no need to rotate the cystoscope in different positions to achieve adequate placement of the laser tip and the prostate. When using videoscopy, the camera can therefore be fixed to the lens of the cystoscope either by direct coupling or by locking the camera head on to the cystoscope lens, as rotation of the cystoscope is not necessary. During videoscopy, rotation of the cystoscope while the camera is in the locked position, especially when the verumontanum cannot be observed, can produce 'disorientation' in the prostatic fossa.

After each quadrant has been lased, the lens and fibre are removed, allowing the bladder to empty. Continuous-flow cystoscopy, or placement of a suprapubic catheter can be used and this obviates routine emptying of the bladder; however, in the author's opinion these techniques are seldom required. During the emptying phase the fibre is meticulously cleaned with a soft cotton bud. If the efficacy of the fibre is in doubt, it may then be checked on the power meter. Thus, cystoscopic deflection and evolving techniques utilizing the cystoscope as an aid in fibre placement during the procedure are critical.

Just before termination of the procedure any areas of haemorrhage can be controlled by 'painting' the area of bleeding. In the canine studies reported by Johnson et al,[4] a ring of thermal damage was noted surrounding the area of coagulative necrosis. Costello has determined that this is actually a zone of arteriolar thrombosis,[7] which accounts for the bloodless nature of the procedure. If bleeding occurs during the procedure this can be controlled either immediately by painting the bleeding point or by continuation with the procedure to its conclusion, thus producing a circumferential ring of thermal damage.

Once the prostate has been lased, the laser fibre is tested on the power meter. The pre- and postoperative power meter readings are then documented in the medical record to prove the efficacy of the laser fibre throughout the procedure. If during lasing there is any question as to the durability of the fibre it should be tested immediately.

An 18 Fr 5 ml Foley catheter is then placed in the bladder. The effluent from the catheter should be essentially clear at the conclusion of the procedure.

Postoperative care

Each patient received intensive pre- and postoperative education concerning what he should expect in the immediate postoperative period, with regard to results of surgery and possible complications, length of catheterization and activity levels. To this end, patients were given educational brochures describing their postoperative course and potential complications. Before discharge from the ambulatory surgery unit all patients were given instructions regarding care of the Foley catheter and leg bag.

All patients were treated with oral antibiotics for 5 days, taking into account their drug allergies and tolerance. When possible, patients were given 800 mg ibuprofen every 8 h for 5 days after operation.

Patients were instructed to remove the Foley catheter on a Monday morning and were asked to report to the office that afternoon to determine their voiding status. Patients were subsequently followed with assessments of AUA-6 symptom score, post-voiding residual urine and peak voiding flowmetry at 1, 6 and 12 months.

Results

All 80 patients were treated as outpatients. The results of assessments at 1, 6 and 12 months are presented in Table 17.1. An average of 5 days were required for Foley catheterization. Four patients required replacement of the Foley catheter with, on average, 2 days catheterization after replacement.

Parameter*	Follow-up period (months)			
	0 (baseline)	1	6	12
No. of patients	80	80	54	16
AUA-6 score	20.8	NA†	7.1	6.5
PVR (ml)	238.5	58.3	50.2	65
Flow (ml/s)	6.3	10.5	14.3	14.8

Table 17.1. Postoperative assessments (1, 6 amd 12 months) of 80 patients receiving visual laser ablation of the prostate

*AUA-6 score, American Urological Association symptom score; PVR, post-voiding residual urine; Flow, peak urine flow rate; †NA, not assessed.

Five patients complained of dysuria requiring urinary analgesics. One patient was noted to have an uncomplicated urinary tract infection without fever.

No patient reported impotence postoperatively who previously had been potent. Of the potent patients, 16% were found to have retrograde ejaculation.

No patient required irrigation of the catheter secondary to sloughed prostatic debris or clot retention. The debris is characterized by a cloudy urine with some pink urethral discharge.

No immediate postoperative complications associated with resorption of fluid were encountered. Patients were instructed to return to normal activity the day following VLAP. They were advised to proceed with intercourse at their discretion, following removal of the Foley catheter.

No surgical procedures were required within the first year of follow-up to relieve either recurrent bladder outlet obstruction or persistent voiding difficulties.

Discussion

Clearly, as shown by the above data, patients who have undergone VLAP achieve a significant improvement in symptom score, post-voiding residual urine and peak flow rate. This improvement is lasting and durable at 1 year follow-up.

If symptoms of bladder outlet obstruction are attributable to residual urine and decreased flow, these results show that there has been a significant improvement at 1 month in both post-voiding residual urine and peak voiding flowmetry. As noted, however, peak flow continues to improve after 1 month and by 6 months has attained a plateau, remaining stable throughout a year. In the author's experience (data not shown), most patients attain normalization of their symptom scores by 1 month postoperatively.

Serious complications that can occur during TURP, such as bleeding and resorption of fluid resulting in hyponatraemia and the TUR syndrome, do not occur with VLAP. This is particularly important in many patients undergoing surgical treatment for the relief of bladder outlet obstruction, because of their advanced age and physical debility. Not only is operative and postoperative haemorrhage important to the patient, it is also increasingly important to the health professional. Long-term complications such as impotence, incontinence and bladder neck contracture or stricture appear to be less likely with VLAP than TURP, when viewed retrospectively. In fact, in this study these complications did not occur. Other adverse events, such as dysuria and uncomplicated urinary tract infection, although annoying are generally easily treated and do not create a significant postoperative problem.

It appears that one compromise associated with this technique is the need to wear a catheter for a few days. However, the incidence of retrograde ejaculation is significantly decreased compared with historical findings associated with TURP. Patients are able to resume normal activity including employment, if desired, immediately after the procedure; this has both economic and social advantages.

Patients should be made aware of the irritative voiding symptoms such as urgency, urgency incontinence and dysuria that may occur following VLAP; these may occur to the same extent in patients who have undergone TURP.[5] In this study, four patients required treatment for their dysuria. Although not identified in this particular patient series, patients may experience the 'post-VLAP syndrome', which consists of prolonged irritative voiding symptoms, especially dysuria, frequency and urgency.

Further study is needed to document the aetiology, incidence and treatment of this uncommon problem.

Although no patients in this series required repeat surgical intervention within the first year of follow-up, this probably will not be a universal finding. Although stricture and bladder neck contracture was not seen in this patient series, with increasing patient numbers these complications will be encountered.

In conclusion, although many questions remain to be answered, this study demonstrates that patients undergoing the VLAP procedure for the relief of bladder outlet obstruction secondary to BPH have significant improvement in both symptoms and objective parameters, which are durable for 1 year. Proper patient selection, surgical technique and patient education are critical for the success of this new technology.

References

1. Holtgrewe H L, Mebust W K, Dowd J B et al. Transurethral prostatectomy: practice aspects of the dominant operation in American urology. J Urol 1989; 141: 248
2. Mebust W K, Holtgrewe H L. Current status of transurethral prostatectomy: a review of the AUA National Cooperative Study. World J Urol 1989; 6: 194
3. Barry M J. Epidemiology and natural history of benign prostatic hyperplasia. Urol Clin North Am 1990; 17: 495
4. Johnson D E, Levinson A K, Greskovich F J, Cromeens D M. Hisopathological changes occurring in the prostate following transurethral laser prostatectomy. In: Anderson R R (ed) Laser surgery: advanced characterization, therapeutics, and systems III SPIE Proc, 1992; 1643: 15–18
5. Cowles R S. Long term follow-up of a prospective randomized trial comparing TURP to VLAP. Presentation, AUA, 1993
6. Barry M J, Fowler F J Jr, O'Leary M P. The American Urological Association symptom index for benign prostatic hyperplasia. J Urol 1992; 148: 1549–1557
7. Costello A J. Personal communication, 1994

Interstitial laser coagulation of benign prostatic hyperplasia: three years' experience

18

R. Muschter   A. P. Perlmutter   S. Hessel   A. Hofstetter

Introduction

Over the last few decades, surgical resection of the prostate, especially the transurethral procedure (TURP), has become the 'gold standard' in the therapy of benign prostatic hyperplasia (BPH). However, despite many surgical and technical improvements, the rate of total morbidity related to TURP has remained approximately 20%.[1-7] A variety of alternative, minimally invasive treatment modalities, therefore, have been (and still are) under investigation. Most recently, thermal energy sources, such as microwaves, radiofrequency waves, high-energy focused ultrasound and lasers, have been tested experimentally and clinically for their ability to destroy prostatic tissue by hyperthermic, coagulative or ablative effects.[8-12]

The new concept of minimally invasive BPH treatment developed by the authors' group[13,14] is based on the creation of voluminous intraprostatic coagulation lesions. In contrast to any heat treatment where energy from a source inside the urethra is delivered to the periurethral prostatic tissue, in interstitial energy delivery the urethra would not be affected. As a consequence there would be no sloughing of necrotic tissue, thus avoiding all related problems, such as irritation. The necrotic material was expected to be resorbed with time, leading to an atrophic, shrunken gland.

In previously published experimental and clinical studies[14-16], the authors demonstrated that these assumptions were correct. Initial in vitro and animal studies with various light guides for interstitial application of neodymium:yttrium aluminium garnet (Nd:YAG) laser radiation showed the production of small carbonized lesions with the use of bare fibres, but of large homogeneous coagulation zones up to 2 cm in diameter with the use of specially designed interstitial thermotherapy (ITT) fibres. Further experiments using such applicators in combination with Nd:YAG and diode lasers resulted in an operative technique suitable for clinical routine in the treatment of symptomatic BPH.

Patients and methods

As radiation source, initially only Nd:YAG lasers (1064 nm) were used: these were the Dornier Fibertome (Germering, Germany) and the Sharplan 3000 (Tel Aviv, Israel). Very recent studies were performed with various diode lasers—the Diomed 25 (Cambridge, UK; 805 nm), the Indigo 830 (Palo Alto, CA, USA; 830 nm) and the Dornier prototype (Germering, Germany; 980 nm). As a result of clinical demands, special software was developed to run automatic power-formatting programs (see below). In addition, for some lasers (the Dornier Fibertome and Indigo 830), optical

(a)

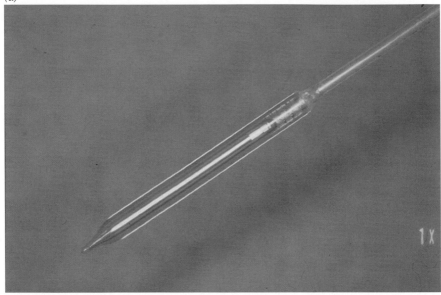

(b)

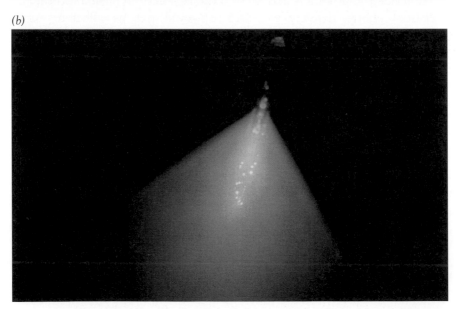

Fig. 18.1. (a) Laser applicator for interstitial laser coagulation (ILC) of the prostate. (b) Conical beam profile (in water).

feedback systems, which in the event of carbonization automatically switch off the system, were developed to avoid thermal fibre damage.

Two types of applicators were employed, a diffuser tip (Sharplan) and a tip with a conical beam pattern (ITT-Light Guide S-6190-1, combined with special adaptor NS/H 6; Dornier) (Fig. 18.1).[17] Both types underwent technical improvements during the clinical tests. Apart from a few variations in the initial phase, all Nd:YAG laser applicators were 20 mm in length and 1.9 mm in diameter. With the diode lasers, several prototypes of light guides, predominantly diffuser tips, were tested. With the 830 nm wavelength, a diffuser tip of 10 mm emitting length and 1.2 mm diameter, made of Teflon (Diffuser-Tip, Indigo), was used almost exclusively.

The tip of the light guide was repeatedly inserted into the prostate either transurethrally through a cystoscope under direct vision (Fig. 18.2) or percutaneously from the perineum under transrectal ultrasound guidance (Fig. 18.3). The number of fibre placements depends on the size and configuration of the gland. On average, 6.2 (range 2–15) fibre placements were made, with a total energy of 21 700 J (2400–48 300 J). Radiation parameters were optimized for each system. To avoid charring, relatively low laser powers and long radiation times (e.g. 7 W for 10 min) or power-formatting programs (e.g. stepwise from 20 to 7 W reduced power for a total of 3 min—'turbo' mode) (Fig. 18.4) were applied.

A suprapubic catheter was inserted routinely in almost every patient before or during treatment. This was intermittently closed from the first postopertaive day to allow the patient to micturate at the earliest stage, and in order to monitor residual urine volumes. Catheters were removed as soon as residual urine volume was less than 50 ml. Usually no transurethral catheter was fitted.

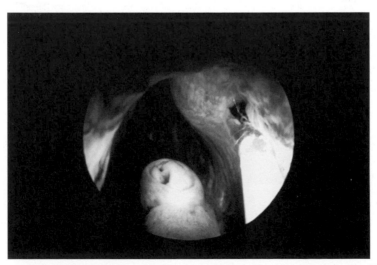

Fig. 18.2. Transurethral application of light guide in ILC. Applicator in situ in the apical left lobe.

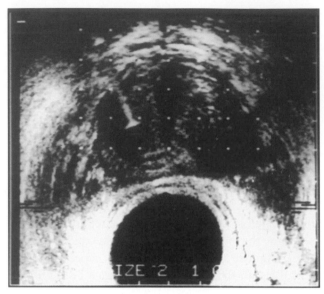

Fig. 18.3. Perineal application of light guide in ILC. Transrectal ultrasound image with aiming grid. Applicator in situ in the right lobe.

From July 1991 to October 1993, 239 patients with BPH (average age 67.8 years; range 48–89 years) with indications for TURP because of obstruction or severe symptoms were treated, who have now completed a 1 year follow-up.

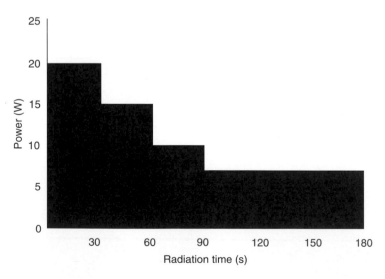

Fig. 18.4. Graphical description of the power-formatting program (stepwise reduced from 20 to 7 W) used with the Nd:YAG laser/ITT light guide in interstitial laser coagulation of the prostate ('turbo' mode). Total radiation time 3 min, total energy 1980 J.

Results

Average American Urological Association (AUA) symptom scores, peak flow rates and residual urine volumes of patients treated with interstitial laser coagulation (ILC) improved substantially from pretreatment to follow-up (all p values <0.001) (Table 18.1). The prostate volume decreased from an average of 47.4 cm^3 (15–175 cm^3) to 32.2 cm^3 after 3 months (approximately 35%).

In the early postoperative period, severe complications were rare (Table 18.2). Most patients experienced a transient exacerbation of urinary flow

Parameter	Follow-up period (months)			
	0 (baseline)	3	6	12
No. of patients	239	239*	216	198
AUA score	25.4 ± 3.9	8.1 ± 6.3	6.1 ± 4.3	6.1 ± 4.2
Urine peak flow (ml/s)	7.7 ± 4.1	16.3 ± 6.9	17.9 ± 7.3	17.8 ± 7.3
Urine residual volume (ml)	151 ± 137	32 ± 56	18 ± 40	19 ± 34
Prostate volume (ml)	47.4 ± 22.1	32.2 ± 15.8	28.2 ± 15.7	29.1 ± 17.1
No. of patients re-treated	—	9*	9 (Σ18)	5 (Σ23)
No. of patients dead/lost to follow-up	—	1*/0	2/2 (Σ5)	0/13 (Σ18)

Table 18.1. Results of follow-up of patients treated with interstitial laser coagulation (ILC) for benign prostatic hyperplasia

*Data collected before re-treatment are included in 3 month values.

Complication	Patients	
	n*	%*
None	156	65.3
Bacteriuria/uncomplicated UTI†	85	35.6
Irritative symptoms/sloughing	30	12.6
Pain	1	0.4
Epididymitis	1	0.4
UTI† with fever	5	2.1
Secondary haemorrhage	5	2.1
With clot retention	3	1.3
With transfusion	1	0.4
Stress incontinence (transient)	1	0.4

Table 18.2. Early complications of ILC of the prostate in 239 patients

*Totals are more than 239 and 100% as some patients had multiple complications; †UTI, urinary trait infection.

and obstructive symptoms (the suprapubic catheter was therefore left in place until the voiding function was sufficient). Few patients (12.6%) suffered irritative symptoms; these were usually accompanied by sloughing of tissue, indicating that the urethra probably was partially included in the necrotic lesion. Uncomplicated urinary tract infections were common; these were significantly less (60 vs 19%, p <0.001) when prophylactic antibiotics (e.g. co-trimoxazole, one single dose per day) were used. One secondary haemorrhage with clot retention requiring blood transfusion stopped after removal of the suprapubic catheter, without further treatment.

Twenty-three patients (9.6%) required re-treatment for persisting or recurrent obstruction or symptoms. Two patients were re-treated within 1 month, seven within months 1–3, nine within months 3–6, and five within months 6–12. Nineteen patients subsequently underwent TURP and one had an open prostatectomy; six patients requested (and received) a second laser treatment (Table 18.3). Reoperation for urethral stricture was necessary in nine (3.8%) and for bladder neck stenosis in four (1.7%) cases.

Erectile function complications were not seen. Of 163 patients who claimed (by questionnaire) to have normal ejaculation prior to laser treatment, 152 (93.3%) reported normal ejaculation at 1 year.

	Patients	
Complication	n*	%*
None	201	84.1
Stricture	13	5.4
BPH surgery†	23	9.6
Other	1	0.4
Unrelated death	3	1.3
Unrelated other	1	0.4

Table 18.3. Late complications of ILC of the prostate in 239 patients
*As in Table 18.2; †second laser treatment, TURP or open prostatectomy.

Discussion

Although this study reports the complete clinical development and learning period of a new procedure in an unselected group of BPH patients, the results compare favourably with those for TURP, as reported by Lepor and Rigaud[18] (peak flow increase from 8.1 to 16.8 ml/s) and Nielsen et al[19] (peak flow increase from 9.5 to 19.6 ml/s), and are similar to, or better than, those of several authors using transurethral ultrasound-guided laser-induced prostatectomy (TULIP)[11,20–24] or visual laser ablation of the prostate (VLAP).[12,24–28]

Few other authors have reported their experiences with ILC using bare fibres or the technique described here.[29–32] McNicholas et al,[29] who treated 15 patients with bare fibres, saw a peak flow increase from 10.0 to 14.4 ml/s. Henkel et al[31] treated 38 patients with perineal ILC and found an AUA score increase from an average of 26 to 9; 50% of their patients experienced a postoperative peak flow rate of 15 ml/s or more. Orovan and Whelan[32] reported an improvement of AUA score from 16.3 to 5.8, of peak flow from 8.8 to 11.9 ml/s and of residual urine volume from 146 to 20 ml in 16 patients treated transurethrally.

Suprapubic catheter times and uncomplicated urinary tract infections after ILC were of the same magnitude as in other laser procedures. After TULIP the suprapubic catheter was left in situ for an average of 11.6–18.1 days,[22–24] after VLAP for an average of 5.7–14 days.[24,26] The rate of urinary tract infections after TULIP was reported to be 18.7–21%.[11,23] Average catheter times following TURP have been reported only infrequently but are probably shorter. The rate of urinary tract infections after TURP is reported as being between 2 and 40%.[4,6]

Significant morbidity, with regard to bleeding and clot retention, which is common in TURP (5.3–19.6%),[3,6,33] is very rare in ILC; regarding the TURP syndrome (0–40%)[4,34] and capsule perforation (1.8%),[33] morbidity may even be described as non-existent after ILC. TURP can affect potency (0–40%)[5,6,35,36] and ejaculation (55–89%).[5,37] In ILC, sexual function is affected in only a few patients. The rate of urethral and bladder neck strictures in this study was of the same magnitude as after TURP[4,5,7,19] and is probably related to the transurethral operation itself, not to the laser application in particular. Compared with other types of laser treatment of BPH in their initial clinical phase, the complication rate of ILC is low.[11,12,20] Mechanical bladder perforation, as seen by Schulze et al[20] in TULIP, did not occur. Persistent urinary incontinence as a consequence of TURP has been reported in the literature in 0.4 to 9%;[3,5,6,33] in the TULIP and VLAP series this occurred only infrequently, and in the study reported here, no patient suffered persistent incontinence. Postoperative irritative symptoms, which frequently occur after TULIP and VLAP (30–85.7%),[11,23,24,26–28] are less likely to appear after ILC (12.6%). As such symptoms after laser-induced ITT were usually connected with tissue sloughing, they probably indicated accidental urethral coagulation. In this case, the effects of ILC were like those of deep transurethral free-beam laser coagulation and were not harmful.

The need for reoperation is more frequent in ILC than in TURP.[1,19] No published information on other laser techniques involves sufficient patients at 1 year follow-up for an accurate assessment of reoperation rates, the exception being Costello's report on 153 patients[26] with a re-treatment rate of 10.5%.

The reduction in volume of the prostate seen after ILC was a mean of 35% and therefore much greater than that seen with most other minimal invasive techniques.[20,23,24,38] Henkel et al[31] reported a volume decrease of 5–48%. Although in the short term the clinical outcome of ILC and TULIP or VLAP[38] is in the same range, in the authors' opinion the marked prostate volume reduction after ILC will positively influence the long-term results and the recurrence rate.

References

1. Melchior J, Valk W L, Foret J D, Mebust W K. Transurethral prostatectomy: computerized analysis of 2,223 consecutive cases. J Urol 1974; 112: 634–642
2. Mebust W K, Holtgrewe H L, Cockett A T K et al. Transurethral prostatectomy: immediate and postoperative complications. A cooperative study of 13 participating institutions evaluating 3,885 patients. J Urol 1989; 141: 243–247
3. Holtgrewe H L, Mebust W K, Dowd J B et al. Transurethral prostatectomy: practice aspects of the dominant operation in American urology. J Urol 1989; 141: 248–253
4. Lewis D C, Burgess N A, Hudd C, Matthews P N. Open or transurethral surgery for the large prostate gland. Br J Urol 1992; 69: 598–602
5. Rollema H J, van Mastrigt R. Improved indication and followup in transurethral resection of the prostate using the computer program CLIM: a prospective study. J Urol 1992; 148: 111–116
6. Doll H A, Black N A, McPherson K et al. Mortality, morbidity and complications following transurethral resection of the prostate for benign prostatic hypertrophy. J Urol 1992; 147: 1566–1573
7. Hammarsten J, Lindqvist K. Suprapubic catheter following transurethral resection of the prostate: a way to decrease the number of urethral strictures and improve the outcome of operations. J Urol 1992; 147: 648–652
8. Devonec M, Ogden C, Perrin P, St Clair Carter S. Clinical response to transurethral microwave thermotherapy is thermal dose dependent. Eur Urol 1993; 23: 267–274
9. Goldwasser B, Ramon J, Engelberg S et al. Transurethral needle ablation (TUNA) of the prostate using low-level radiofrequency energy: an animal experimental study. Eur Urol 1993; 24: 400–405
10. Marberger M, Madersbacher S, Kratzik C. Treatment of BPH by thermal ablation with transrectal high-intensity focused ultrasound (HIFU). J Urol 1993; 149: 217A
11. McCullough D L, Assimos D G, Harrison L H. TULIP—transurethral ultrasound guided laser induced prostatectomy—sequential depiction of prostatic urethral laser induced changes from the pre-operative state to 32 weeks post-operatively. J Urol 1992; 147(suppl): 210A
12. Costello A J, Bowsher W G, Bolton D M et al. Laser ablation of the prostate in patients with benign prostatic hypertrophy. Br J Urol 1992; 69: 603–608
13. Hofstetter A. Interstitielle Thermokoagulation (ITK) von Prostatatumoren. Lasermedizin 1991; 7: 179
14. Muschter R, Hofstetter A, Hessel S et al. Hi-tech of the prostate: interstitial laser coagulation of benign prostatic hypertrophy. In: Anderson R R (ed) Laser surgery: advanced characterization, therapeutics, and systems III. SPIE Proc 1992; 1643: 25–34
15. Muschter R, Hofstetter A, Hessel S et al. Interstitial laser prostatectomy—experimental and first clinical results. J Urol 1992; 147(suppl); 346A
16. Muschter R, Hessel S, Hofstetter A et al. Die interstitielle Laserkoagulation der benignen Prostatahyperplasie. Urologie [A] 1993; 32: 273–281
17. Hessel S, Frank F. Technical prerequisites for the interstitial thermo-therapy using the Nd:YAG laser. In: Katzir A (ed) Optical fibers in medicine V. SPIE Proc 1990; 1201: 233–238
18. Lepor H, Rigaud G. The efficacy of transurethral resection of the prostate in men with moderate symptoms of prostatism. J Urol 1990; 143: 533–537
19. Nielsen K T, Christensen M M, Madsen P O, Bruskewitz R C. Symptom analysis and uroflowmetry 7 years after transurethral resection of the prostate. J Urol 1989; 142: 1251–1253

20. Schulze H, Martin W, Engelmann U, Senge T. TULIP—transurethrale ultraschallgeführte laserinduzierte Prostatektomie: eine Alternative zur TURP? Urologe [A] 1993; 32: 225–231

21. McCullough D L, Roth R A, Babayan R K et al. Transurethral ultrasound-guided laser-induced prostatectomy: National Human Cooperative Study results. J Urol 1993; 150: 1607–1611

22. Takahashi S, Homma Y, Minowada S, Aso Y. Transurethral ultrasound-guided laser-induced prostatectomy (TULIP) for benign prostatic hyperplasia: clinical utility at one-year follow-up and imaging analysis. Urology 1994; 43: 802–808

23. Puppo P, Perachino M, Ricciotti G, Scannapieco G. Transurethral ultrasound-guided laser-induced prostatectomy. Objective and subjective assessment of its efficacy for treating benign prostatic hyperplasia. Eur Urol 1994; 25: 220–225

24. De la Rosette J J M C H, Froeling F M J A, Alivizatos G, Debruyne F M J. Laser ablation of the prostate: experience with an ultrasound guided technique and a procedure under direct vision. Eur Urol 1994; 25: 19–24.

25. Kabalin J N. Laser prostatectomy performed with a right angle firing neodymium:YAG laser fiber at 40 watts power setting. J Urol 1993; 150: 95–99

26. Costello A J. Evolving experience in treatment of benign prostatic obstruction using Nd:YAG laser at St Vincent's Hospital, Melbourne. Aust NZ J Surg 1995; in press.

27. Shanberg A M, Lee I S, Tansey L A, Sawyer D E. Extensive neodymium-YAG photoirradiation of the prostate in men with obstructive prostatism. Urology 1994; 43: 467–471

28. Cowles R S. Results after nine months of a prospective randomized study comparing transurethral resection of the prostate and visual laser ablation of the prostate. In: Lasers in urology, gynecology, and general surgery SPIE Proc 1993; 1879: 76–78

29. McNicholas T A, Aslam M, Lynch M J, O'Donoghue N. Interstitial laser coagulation for the treatment of urinary outflow obstruction. J Urol 1993; 149: 465A

30. Hoopes J P, Williams J C, Harris R D et al. Interstitial laser coagulation (ILC) of the canine prostate with transrectal ultrasound (TRUS) and thermal monitoring. J Urol 1994; 151: 334A

31. Henkel T O, Greschner M, Luppold T et al. Perineal interstitial laser of the prostate (PILP). SPIE Proc 1994; 2327: in press

32. Orovan W L, Whelan J P. Neodymium YAG laser treatment of BPH using interstitial thermotherapy: a transurethral approach. J Urol 1994; 151: 230A

33. Edwards L E, Bucknall T E, Pittam M R et al. Transurethral resection of the prostate and bladder neck incision: a review of 700 cases. Br J Urol 1985; 57: 168–171

34. Goel C M, Badenoch D F, Fowler C G et al. Transurethral resection syndrome. A prospective study. Eur Urol 1992; 21: 15–17

35. Lue T F. Impotence after prostatectomy. Urol Clin North Am 1990; 17: 613–620

36. Samdal F, Vada K, Lundmo P. Sexual function after transurethral prostatectomy. Scand J Urol Nephrol 1993; 27: 27–29

37. Lindner A, Golomb J, Korzcak D et al. Effects of prostatectomy on sexual function. Urology 1991; 38: 26–28

38. Muschter R, Zellner M, Hofstetter A. Lasers and benign prostatic hyperplasia—experimental and clinical results to compare different application systems. J Urol 1994; 151: 230A

Laser ablation of the prostate: coagulation versus vaporization

19

J. J. M. C. H. de la Rosette

Introduction

Benign prostatic hyperplasia (BPH) is one of the most common diseases in men, and its impact on medical care is increasing due to the ageing of the population and changes in social habits. The majority of men will eventually experience some voiding symptoms due to BPH and a significant minority will seek surgical therapy during their lifetime.

The treatment of BPH is currently undergoing significant re-evaluation. Because of the medical and economic impact of prostate surgery, a number of alternatives to traditional transurethral resection of the prostate (TURP) have emerged during the past few years. One alternative to TURP that recently demonstrated significant results is the use of lasers in prostatectomy.

Laser light is a unique form of energy with characteristic and variable tissue effects. When the laser beam hits the tissue, approximately 60–70% of energy is absorbed and 30–40% is reflected. In the non-contact mode the major part of depth penetration is due to forward diffusion. The depth of tissue penetration of the laser beam is theoretically 4–8 mm.[1] Moreover, energy conversion to heat depends on the type of tissue treated, specifically its composition and vascularity. Prostatic tissue heated to 60–100°C will undergo protein denaturation and coagulation necrosis. Visually, the denatured prostatic tissue will appear blanched yet remain intact. Coagulation results in delayed sloughing of the prostate for a variable period, usually several weeks after the procedure. At temperatures above 100°C, tissues become vapours of water and hydrocarbons, thus creating immediate cavitation.

Additional factors beyond wavelength influence tissue effects. Increasing the energy density can also alter the tissue effects. This can be accomplished by a change in the power output or in the duration of application of the laser beam. Alteration in the amount of power for a given area of tissue, that is the laser spot size, significantly changes the energy density and tissue effects. Increasing the energy density by bringing the laser fibre tip into contact with the tissue decreases the spot size, increases the tissue temperature, and improves the vaporizing characteristics of a neodymium:yttrium aluminium garnet (Nd:YAG) laser.[2]

The first published report of laser treatment of BPH was that by Johnson et al.[1] Subsequently various authors have reported their clinical experiences in humans using different types of applicators.[3–8] These applicators, however, differ in their physical properties, overall performance and tissue effects.

Which type of applicator to use is a fundamental question. In favour of a vaporizing technique is the fact that tissue is vaporized and a lumen created instantly, there is minimal postoperative oedema and a lower incidence of postoperative urinary retention, especially in large glands. On the other hand, a greater depth of penetration is achieved by coagulation, resulting in more extensive tissue destruction which thus should lead to wider prostatic urethral opening with better urine flow rates. Until now, no long-term data have been available to demonstrate this correlation with clinical results in humans. A study therefore conducted using a fibre primarily used to achieve coagulation (Urolase®) and a fibre to achieve vaporization (Ultraline®). The results are reported here together with an overview of the available literature.

Personal experience

The author's initial experience with laser treatment of BPH were with the transurethral ultrasound-guided laser-induced prostatectomy (TULIP®) device and the Urolase fibre.[9] However, the simplicity of the endoscopic-assisted technique made it more attractive than the ultrasound-guided TULIP device. Moreover, the latter procedure caused more morbidity.

This experience was followed by use of the side-firing fibre technique. In a randomized fashion 90 patients were treated with the Ultraline® fibre (Heraeus) and the Urolase® fibre (Bard). The Urolase fibre aims at deep coagulation whereas the Ultraline fibre enables vaporization. The Ultraline® fibre was used at a 60 W setting, 'painting' the prostate, and the Urolase® fibre was used at a 40 W setting for 90 s at predetermined areas. The techniques used have been described by several authors in more detail.[5,10] Before the laser therapy, patients were assessed with the International Prostate Symptom Score (IPSS). Other investigations included a digital rectal examination, transrectal ultrasonography of the prostate, a renal ultrasound examination, urethrocystoscopy, uroflowmetry and pressure flow studies, urine culture and cytology, and routine blood studies, including prostate-specific antigen (PSA) determination.

The prostate volumes ranged from 26 to 83 cm³ (average 45.3 cm³) in the Ultraline® group and from 29 to 76 cm³ (average 50.2 cm³) in the Urolase® group. Twelve weeks after treatment, the mean symptom score in the Ultraline® group fell from 21.2 (SD±6.0) to 8.0 (±5.0) and the mean peak flow increased from 7.8 (±2.9) to 19.1 (±7.2) ml/s. In the Urolase® group, the symptom score improved from 21.1 (±5.1) to 8.1 (±5.5) with a peak flow improvement from 7.9 ($\pm$3.0) to 19.5 ($\pm$6.8) ml/s. In both groups there was a signficant decrease in post-voiding residual urine and the suprapubic catheter was needed for an average of 2–3 weeks. Morbidity, consisting of irritative complaints, was seen in both groups at the same rate and severity.

Discussion

By almost any subjective measurement of symptom score, or objective assessment such as change in flow rate, TURP still provides results that are superior to alternative forms of therapy and remains the standard for comparison with new technologies. The advantages and ultimate acceptance of new technology rely, as well as on results comparable to those with TURP, upon improvements in treatment-related morbidity. With laser therapy, most opportunities seem to lie in the possibility of decreased bleeding, shorter hospitalization and a reduced requirement of anaesthesia.

The author's initial experience with the TULIP device was very encouraging. However, the procedure appeared to be cumbersome and the morbidity was considerable.[9] In fact, obstructive and irritative symptoms in most patients were aggravated and increased immediately after the procedure, probably because of laser-related oedema and local tissue response. These findings have been confirmed by other authors.[4,11,12]

The non-contact side-firing laser technology has made the procedure user friendly and time efficient for all urologists. A significant difference between laser prostatectomy and standard TURP is the lack of immediacy of effect. A standard TURP removes tissue at the time of the procedure and patients often experience a significant improvement in urinary stream as soon as the Foley catheter is removed. There is some immediate surface tissue vaporization with the Nd:YAG laser during laser prostatectomy but the key to the success of this procedure is the deeper tissue ablation by means of coagulation necrosis, followed by a much slower slough of the affected BPH. As experience of side-fire coagulation has grown, it has become apparent that some patients require prolonged periods of catheter drainage postoperatively. To be accepted as an altenative to TURP, successful early catheter removal within 24 h of the visual laser ablation of the prostate (VLAP) procedure, without signficant morbidity, is required. Vaporization appears to allow the earlier removal of catheters and reduction in postoperative discomfort.[13]

Shanberg and associates were among the first to describe a method for laser prostatectomy wherein an end-fire Nd:YAG laser fibre was placed in direct contact with the prostatic tissue.[14] The prostate can be vaporized, instead of coagulated. This can be achieved either by using a higher power density than that used for coagulation or by using a wavelength that is absorbed better. Contact laser prostatectomy is only one way of achieving vaporization. Sapphire-tip probes have been developed as a more effective method for direct contact vaporization of tissue. The contact of the delivery system with the tissue results in a higher power density than is usually achieved with a free-beam approach. In addition, the contact tip may be coated with an infrared absorber or it may become slightly coated with carbon after contact with the tissue. This therefore increases the absorption and promotes a tendency to vaporize the tissue.

Until now, the primary limitation has been that, even with some of the design changes and improvements, vaporization of the prostate has been relatively slow and tedious, especially when a large amount of tissue is involved.[2] Contact laser treatment of the prostate theoretically is appealing because the technique results in immediate tissue vaporization; thus, therapeutic results do not depend upon secondary tissue slough. The immediate voiding problems experienced by some patients after non-contact laser treatment methods may be avoided with contact lasers. In view of the limitations of the present contact probes, new improvements are awaited, to continue to increase the efficiacy of energy transmission. This should markedly shorten treatment duration of the future.

Side-firing fibres also have been used for vaporization. Narayan et al have presented their results, using the Ultraline® fibre. The main findings of their study, were that transurethral evaporation of the prostate, in the short term, provides symptomatic relief and improvement in urine flow comparable to that with TURP.[5] However, the present author could not confirm this observation when using the Ultraline® fibre for laser treatment, concluding that a significant reduction in symptom scores and improvement in peak urine flow can be achieved with both fibres used and that the results obtained with both fibres are comparable. The vaporization technique (using the Ultraline® fibre), which might have been expected to result in an earlier recovery of adequate spontaneous micturition and diminution of the symptoms, did not, in fact, do so. It is possible that the technique used with this type of fibre does not achieve optimum vaporization. Evaporation of tissue is favoured by high power density and to obtain maximal power density, it is important to maintain the fibre in close contact with the tissue. As this was not achieved in the present study this may explain why evaporation was less than expected. The main reason for not working in constant contact was because it had been assumed that the fibres would deteriorate more rapidly if used in this way. The effect of the Ultraline® fibre, at least when used as described above for the present study, is probably, therefore, the result of both coagulation and vaporization.

Finally, interstitial laser coagulation is another interesting treatment option performed with a specially designed applicator system. These

Technique	Authors	Fibre/procedure	No. of patients	Q_{max} (ml/s) before surgery and at follow-up*			
				0 (baseline)	3	6	12
Vaporization							
Contact	Watson et al[8]	SLT contact fibre	24	6.4	18.0	19.4	—
Non-contact	Narayan et al[5]	Ultraline	61	9.3	15.5	13.2	24.6
	de la Rosette[†]	Ultraline	43	7.8	19.5	14.5	16.2
Coagulation							
Interstitial	Muschter et al[7]	ITT[‡]	239	7.7	16.3	17.7	17.6
Non-contact	Leach et al[15]	Urolase	28	8.1	12.8	13.0	—
	Kabalin[16]	Urolase	190	6.7	14.8	16.4	18.5
	Norris et al[17]	Urolase	108	7.5	—	12.0	—
	Anson and Watson[18]	Urolase	23	9.7	23.0	21.0	20.0
	de la Rosette[†]	Urolase	47	7.8	19.5	14.5	—
	Leach et al[19]	Urolase	117	7.4	—	14.3	16.0
	Buckley et al[20]	Urolase	77	9.9	—	17.5	—
	Costello and Crowe[21]	Urolase	35	8.7	14.4	15.7	20.8
	Takahashi et al[4]	TULIP	30	7.6	13.9	—	14.7
	McCullough and Schulze[12]	TULIP	72	6.5	17.2	19.7	19.1
	Boon et al[11]	TULIP	211	7.4	12.3	12.3	11.6
	Anson and Watson[18]	Myriadlase	23	9.5	12.8	15.9	13.5

Table 19.1. Changes in peak urinary flow rate (Q_{max}) after laser ablation of the prostate

*0=baseline; 3, 6 and 12=3, 6 and 12 month follow-up; †personal experience, as reported in this chapter; ‡ITT, interstitial thermotherapy.

Technique	Authors	Fibre/procedure	No. of patients	IPSS values before surgery and at follow-up*			
				0 (baseline)	3	6	12
Vaporization							
Contact	Watson et al[8]	SLT contact fibre	24	22.6	6.0	8.1	—
Non-contact	Narayan et al[5]	Ultraline	61	27.5	8.0	6.6	8.0
	de la Rosette†	Ultraline	43	21.2	8.0	6.9	7.4
Coagulation							
Interstitial	Muschter et al[7]	ITT†‡	239	25.4	8.1	6.4	6.2
Non-contact	Leach et al[15]	Urolase	28	21.0	10.3	9.4	—
	Kabalin[16]	Urolase	190	20.4	10.4	9.2	7.6
	Norris et al[17]	Urolase	108	22.3	—	9.2	—
	Anson and Watson[18]	Urolase	23	19.3	9.5	10.0	7.7
	de la Rosette†	Urolase	47	21.1	8.1	8.1	—
	Leach et al[19]	Urolase	117	21.0	—	8.6	8.3
	Buckley et al[20]	Urolase	77	19.0	—	6.0	—
	Costello and Crowe[21]	Urolase	35	19.9	10.3	8.8	7.3
	Takahashi et al[4]	TULIP	30	22.8	8.0	—	6.2§
	McCullough and Schulze[12]	TULIP	72	17.7	5.4	—	3.2§
	Boon et al[11]	TULIP	227	18.3	7.6	6.9	6.7§
	Anson and Watson[18]	Myriadlase	23	20.5	8.0	8.2	8.1

Table 19.2. International Prostate Symptom Score (IPSS) results after laser ablation of the prostate

*, †, ‡As in Table 19.1; § Boyarsky symptom score.

applicators are inserted in the prostatic tissue, and the procedure causes voluminous intraprostatic coagulation necroses, leading to degeneration and atrophy associated with substantial shrinking of the adenoma. The urethra is usually unaffected. Neither irritative symptoms of importance, nor any sloughing of tissue after treatment, have been observed so far. Interstitial laser coagulation appears to be at least as effective as transurethral laser coagulation of the prostate (when using side-firing fibres), avoiding most of the disadvantages of this procedure.

The results of changes in symptom score and voiding parameters are presented in Tables 19.1 and 19.2.

Conclusions

Recently, a number of new therapeutic approaches to the treatment of symptomatic BPH have emerged. It is important to recognize that the term 'laser prostatectomy' encompasses a wide variety of instruments, laser wavelengths and techniques. Promising results or advantages with one particular method of laser prostatectomy may not be applicable to other techniques. Each laser fibre has its own advantages and limitations, and no single formula exists for the ideal VLAP. The next generation of laser fibres may combine contact and non-contact options more effectively to permit both deep coagulation and adequate creation of a channel through vaporization.

References

1. Johnson D E, Levinson A K, Greskovich F J et al. Transurethural laser prostatectoy using a wide angle delivery system. SPIE Proc 1991; 1421: 36–41
2. Smith J A Jr. Laser treatment of the urethra and prostate. Semin Urol 1991; 3: 180–184
3. Shanberg A M, Lee I S, Tansey L A, Sawyer D E. Extensive neodymium–YAG photoirradiation of the prostate in men with obstructive prostatism. Urology 1994; 43: 467–471
4. Takahashi S, Homma Y, Minowada S, Aso Y. Transurethral ultrasound guided laser induced prostatectomy (TULIP) for benign prostatic hyperplasia: clinical utility at one-year follow up and imaging analysis. Urology 1994; 43: 802–808
5. Narayan P, Fournier G, Indudhara R et al. Transurethral evaporation of prostate (TUEP) with Nd:YAG laser using a contact free beam technique: results in 61 patients with benign prostatic hyperplasia. Urology 1994; 43: 813–820
6. Costello A J, Bowsher W G, Bolton D M et al. Laser ablation of the prostate in patients with benign prostatic hypertrophy. Br J Urol 1992; 69: 603–608
7. Muschter R, Zellner M, Hessel S, Hofstetter A. Lasers and benign prostatic hyperplasia—experimental and clinical results to compare different application systems. J Urol 1994; 151: 230A
8. Watson G, Anson K, Janetschek G et al. An indepth evaluation of contact laser vaporisation of the prostate. J Urol 1994; 151: 231A
9. de la Rosette J J M C H, Froeling F M J A, Alivizatos G, Debruyne F M J. Laser ablation of the prostate: experience with an ultrasound guided technique and a procedure under direct vision. Eur Urol 1994; 25: 19–24
10. Kabalin J N. Laser prostatectomy performed with a right angle firing neodymium:YAG laser fiber at 40 watts power setting. J Urol 1993; 150: 95–99
11. Boon T A, Lepor H, Muschter R, McCullough D L. Laser treatment of benign prostatic

hyperplasia (BPH): workshop in benign prostatic hyperplasia. In: Kurth K, Newling DWW (eds) Benign prostatic hyperplasia—recent progress in clinical research and practice. New York: Wiley-Liss, 1994: 535–544

12. McCullough D L, Schulze H. Transurethral ultrasound guided laser induced prostatectomy (TULIP): US cooperative study and University of Bochum results. In: Kurth K, Newling D W W (eds) Benign prostatic hyperplasia—recent progress in clinical research and practice. New York: Wiley-Liss, 1994: 529–533
13. Anson K, Watson G, Shah T, Barnes D. Laser prostatectomy: our initial experience of a technique in evolution. J Endourol 1993; 7: 333–336
14. Shanberg A M, Tansey C A, Baghdassarian R. The use of Nd:YAG laser in prostatectomy. J Urol 1985; 133: 331A
15. Leach G E, Sirls L, Ganabathi K et al. Outpatient visual laser-assisted prostatectomy under local anesthesia. Urology 1994; 43: 149–153
16. Kabalin J N. Visual laser treatment of BPH: how I do it. Seminar—Lasers in Urologic Practice, AUA Meeting 1994
17. Norris J P, Norris D M, Lee R D, Rubenstein M A. Visual laser ablation of the prostate: clinical experience in 108 patients. J Urol 1993; 150: 1612–1614
18. Anson K M, Watson G. Lasers in the treatment of benign prostatic hyperplasia. In: Puppo P (ed) Contemporary BPH management. Bologna: Monduzzi Editore, 1993: 91–101
19. Leach G E, Dmochowski R, Ganabathi K et al. Visual laser assisted prostatectomy (VLAP) using urolase right angle fiber: multicenter 60 watt protocol. J Urol 1994; 151: 228A
20. Buckley J F, Ligam V, Paterson P. Endoscopic laser ablation of the prostate gland (ELAP). J Urol 1994; 151: 229A
21. Costello A J, Crowe H R. A single institution experience of reflecting laser fibre prostatectomy over four years. J Urol 1994; 151: 229A

Retrograde transurethral KTP-532 laser ablation of posterior urethral valves in neonates, infants and children

20

A. M. Shanberg   D. Hald   A. Khim

Introduction

Posterior urethral valves represent the most common cause of lower urinary tract obstruction in male children. The congenital obstruction of the prostatic urethra can have profound effects on the entire urinary system. Subsequently, a number of techniques for the management of posterior urethral valves have been described in the urological literature. In neonates, the fear of complications from early valve ablation has led many paediatric urologists to perform primary cutaneous vesicostomy and defer surgical correction to allow for growth of the male urethra.[1]

Advances in laser technology and the development of smaller paediatric instrumentation have facilitated the clinical applications of lasers to paediatric urology. Indeed, the use of the neodymium:yttrium aluminium garnet (Nd:YAG) laser in the treatment of congenital valves has been reported previously.[2,3] Ideally, posterior urethral valves are treated with minimal urethral damage and preservation of continence, antegrade ejaculation and renal function. Minimizing the number of operative procedures in this patient population is also desirable. The KTP-532 laser has thermal characteristics optimally suited for posterior urethral valve ablation in the delicate neonatal urethra. In this chapter, the authors' technique and experience in the retrograde, transurethral management of posterior valves in the paediatric population is presented.

Patients and methods

Between 1987 and 1993, 12 patients underwent transurethral KTP-532 laser ablation of posterior urethral valves and have been followed for a minimum of 1 year and a maximum of 6 years. Patient age ranged from 2 days to 7 years. Seven of these children were treated in the first 2 weeks of life and the remainder at ages ranging from 18 months to 7 years (Table 20.1). In five cases, the diagnosis was suspected after prenatal ultrasonography. All neonates with a presumptive diagnosis of posterior urethral valves were initially treated with primary bladder drainage by a 5 Fr feeding tube and empirical antibiotic cover. Radiographic work-up included

197

Child no.	Weight	Age at surgery	Follow-up (years)	Eventual renal function	Comment
1	35 lb (1600 g)	3 years	4	Azotaemia, had ureterostomies at birth	Valve bladder needs intermittent catheterization
2	19 lb (860 g)	8 months	3	Excellent	Residual mild upper tract dilatation
3	1800 g	11 days	3	Excellent	7.2 Fr uretero-scope used
4	2200 g	4 days	2.5	Azotaemia at birth; normal renal function at 1 year	Residual mild upper tract dilatation
5	24 lb (1100 g)	14 months	2	Azotaemia at birth; normal renal function at birth, when treated	Had temporary vesicostomy at birth taken down when valve treated
6	2100 g	10 days	4	Normal at 1 year	Upper tract dilatation 90% resolved
7	2200 g	5 days	4	Normal	Upper tract dilatation resolved
8	2400 g	3 days	VCUG* normal 5 days	Lost to follow-up	
9	30 lb (1400 g)	10 months	2	Massive hydro-nephrosis at birth, resolved with vesicostomy	Mild upper tract dilatation, no hydro-nephrosis
10	Unknown	7 years	6	Normal one dead kidney	Had valve in-completely resected elsewhere at birth
11	1800 g	2 days	1	Normal	
12	Unknown	7 years	2	Normal	Presented only with total incontinence, now resolved

Table 20.1. Data of 12 children undergoing transurethral KTP-532 laser ablation of posterior urethral valves

*VCUG, voiding cystourethrogram.

ultrasonography and voiding cystourethrography in all cases (Fig. 20.1a) and nuclear renal scans or intravenous pyelograms when clinically indicated. In three cases, the endoscopic KTP-532 laser valve ablation was performed as a secondary procedure following simultaneous closure of cutaneous vesicostomy in two cases, and takedown of bilateral uretero-stomies in another child. The smallest patients treated by the authors to date have been two 1800 g neonates treated at 2 and 11 days of life.

Operative technique

After initial medical stabilization and appropriate radiographic work-up, all patients underwent a general anaesthetic with perioperative antibiotic cover. Patients were positioned in the modified lithotomy position and the urethra was generously lubricated with water-soluble anaesthetic gel. In all but the smallest neonate, the 9.2 Fr Olympus cystoscope passed without difficulty, although the meatus had to be dilated frequently with paediatric sounds to 10 Fr size. In the smallest neonate, an ACMI 7.2 Fr short ureteroscope was used for the endoscopic delivery of the laser fibre. A 0.025 mm guide wire was uniformly positioned in the bladder to maintain anatomical orientation. In all cases video cystourethroscopy confirmed the diagnosis of posterior urethral valves and the dual-purpose Nd:YAG/KTP-532 Laserscope (Santa Clara, CA, USA) system was the laser source. The power settings ranged from 2 to 4 W in a continuous-wave mode. Using a 0 degree lens, either a 200 or 400 μm quartz laser fibre was manipulated through the working channel and with video assistance the laser fibre was positioned directly on a valve leaflet (Fig. 20.2). Continuous warm-water irrigation was used and the valves were vaporized in a systematic fashion precisely at the 2, 5, 7 and 11 o'clock positions. Subsequently, cystoscopic examination of the bladder neck and verumontanum showed no evidence of injury and the cystoscope was removed. Utilizing the Seldinger tech-nique, a 6 or 8 Fr silastic urethral catheter was positioned in the bladder and placed to gravity drainage for 24 or 48 h. A pull-out voiding cysto-urethrogram was then performed to confirm valve ablation (Fig. 20.1b).

Results

All 12 children demonstrated radiographic evidence of complete valve ablation. One child required postoperative intermittent catheterization for what is presumed to be a valve bladder. Two children eventually under-went laparoscopic nephrectomy for non-functioning kidneys and one child required ureteral patch augmentation cystoplasty for a poorly compliant valve bladder.

There were no cases of perioperative urinary tract infection or bleeding requiring catheter irrigation. With a mean follow-up of 3.0 years, no ure-thral strictures have been observed. All children are now voiding with a

(a)

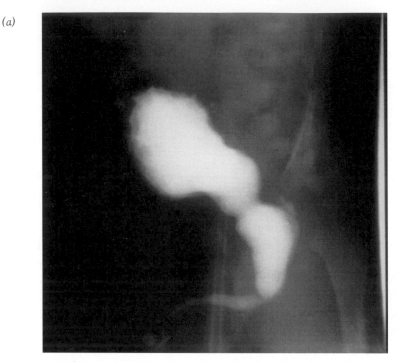

Fig. 20.1. Voiding cystourethrograms (a) demonstrating urethral valve, and (b) (opposite) after operation.

normal urinary stream and no incontinence in the older patients has been observed. Two of the older children have persistent enuresis, but no daytime wetting.

Upper tract dilatation improved in ten of the 12 patients as determined by follow-up renal scans or ultrasonography. One child has poor renal function and will most certainly require renal transplantation. Another patient has a solitary kidney and persistent dilatation of the remaining upper tract, but has no evidence of obstruction on the washout renal scan or Whitaker test. The mean operative time was 30 min for KTP-532 laser valve vaporization.

Discussion

The treatment of paediatric posterior urethral valves challenges the urologist with many management problems. Historically, the management of posterior urethral valves in neonates and infants has had proponents of electrocautery fulguration or resection, avulsion techniques or temporary cutaneous vesicostomy.[4-7] Early experience with the electrothermic manipulation of valves resulted in urethral stricture rates of 50% in children less than 1 year of age.[8] With the development of smaller instrumentation, results in recently published series utilizing electrocautery have yielded stricture rates of 1–8%.[9]

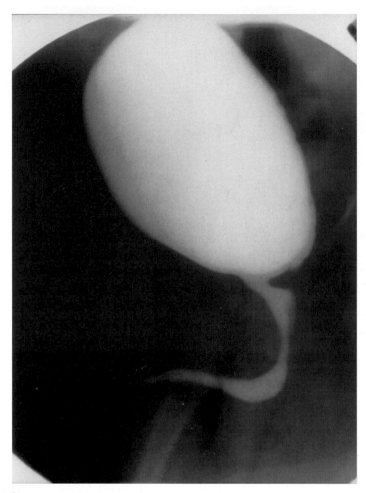

Fig. 20.1(b)

In the early 1980s, Shanberg, Chalfin and Tansey became interested in the use of the Nd:YAG laser in the treatment of recurrent urethral strictures in adults.[10] On the basis of their early experience with the successful management of these recurrent strictures, the application of medical lasers in the treatment of paediatric urethral pathology became conceptually attractive. In 1987, Ehrlich, Shanberg and Fine reported the first use of lasers in the treatment of posterior urethral valves in children.[3] In their original series all patients had prior diverting cutaneous vesicostomy and the valves were treated in an antegrade fashion through the previously established vesicostomy, with subsequent closure of the vesicostomy to prevent scarring of the valve area due to a lack of urinary flow. Non-touch Nd:YAG, sapphire tip Nd:YAG and direct contact KTP-532 laser techniques were used. In their series, no cases of urethral stricture or incontinence were reported.

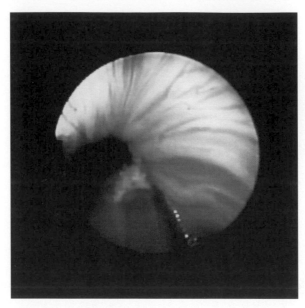

Fig. 20.2. Cystoscopic view of urethral valve.

More recently, Biewald and Schier have reported their experience with the retrograde Nd:YAG laser treatment of urethral valves in neonates.[2] They also have not observed treatment failures or urethral strictures, as has been reported in the electrocautery series. The present authors agree with their conclusion that the medical laser is a safe and reliable method for early management of this difficult problem.

Nevertheless, the KTP-532 laser has several theoretical advantages over the Nd:YAG laser in the confines of the neonatal urethra. Specifically, light at this wavelength has more of a cutting effect and better haemostatic properties, thereby allowing excellent visualization during valve vaporization. In addition, the depth of penetration with the KTP-532 laser is 1–2 mm as opposed to 2–4 mm with the Nd:YAG, with less forward scatter of energy, thereby protecting the surrounding vital structures.[11] Using the KTP-532 laser in a direct touch technique allows for the precise ablation of valve tissue with no bleeding and less trauma to adjacent tissues. In the authors' opinion, the use of the KTP-532 laser in the treatment of valves in children will result in preservation of ejaculatory function in adult life analagous to the results observed in the application of lasers in the treatment of benign prostatic hyperplasia in adults.[12]

The present series started when smaller cystoscopic instrumentation that allowed the passage of a 200 or 400 μm laser fibre through the working channel became available. The ability to manage the neonate effectively with primary valve ablation has avoided vesicostomy in many of these patients. Obviously, there have been cost savings with a single procedure and bladder function has been rapidly restored, which is conceptually attractive. In the light of a recent report by Walker and Padron, that initial diverting vesicostomy offered no long-term advantage over primary valve ablation with respect to ultimate renal function,[7] the retrograde, transurethral KTP-532 laser ablation of valves in patients with mild to moderate degree of renal insufficiency is, in the authors' opinion, the treatment of choice for managing this form of congenital outflow obstruction.

In the follow-up no complications were seen as a consequence of early valve treatment. These data are encouraging, but enthusiasm, as in many areas of paediatric surgery, must be tempered as the ultimate long-term results with respect to continence and ejaculatory function will require many years of follow-up. This modality of therapy offers relative safety in the treatment of this difficult problem in children and the retrograde treatment avoids the staged procedure of temporary cutaneous vesicostomy followed by valve ablation. With the widespread availability of laser technology to the medical community, the definitive endoscopic laser treatment of posterior urethral valves may now be easily performed in a technically satisfying method without risk of serious complication.

References

1. Krueger R P, Hardy B E, Churchill B M. Growth in boys with posterior urethral valves—primary valve resection vs upper tract diversion. Urol Clin North Am 1985; 7: 265
2. Biewald W, Schier F. Laser treatment of posterior urethral valves in neonates. Br J Urol 1992; 69: 425
3. Ehrlich M R, Shanberg A M, Fine R N. Neodymium:YAG laser ablation of urethral valves. J Urol 1987; 138: 959
4. Glassberg K I. Current issues regarding posterior urethral valves in neonates. Urol Clin North Am 1985; 12: 175
5. Whitaker R H, Sherwood T. An improved hook for destroying posterior urethral valves. J Urol 1986; 135: 531
6. Mohan K A. Mohan's urethral valvotome: a new instrument. J Urol 1990; 144: 1196
7. Walker R D, Padron M. The management of posterior urethral valves by initial vesicostomy and delayed valve ablation. J Urol 1990; 144: 1212
8. Myers D A, Walker R D. Prevention of urethral strictures in the management of posterior urethral valves. J Urol 1981; 126: 655
9. Crooks K K. Urethral strictures following the transurethral resection of posterior urethral valves. J Urol 1982; 127: 1153
10. Shanberg A M, Chalfin S A, Tansey L A. Neodymium:YAG laser: new treatment for urethral stricture disease. Urology 1984; 24: 15
11. Stein B S. Laser–tissue interaction. In: Smith J A, Stein B S, Benson R C (eds) Lasers in urologic surgery, 3rd ed. St Louis: Mosby Year Book, 1994; 10–25
12. Leach G E, Sirls L, Ganabathi K et al. Outpatient visual laser-assisted prostatectomy under local anesthesia. Urology 1994; 43: 149

Lasers in benign conditions

21

A. J. Costello

Introduction

Urological surgery has undergone dramatic changes and, like other surgical disciplines, has been swept along on the surge of new technology. The application of this new technology is designed to produce an efficacy equivalent to that of the conventional procedure, but with reduced patient morbidity and increased patient comfort. Shock wave lithotripsy and laparoscopic surgery have already had remarkable impact in the provision of urological surgery since their introduction.

The neodymium:yttrium aluminium garnet (Nd:YAG) laser was first used in the treatment of prostatic disease in the early 1980s. The attempts to ablate adenoma using end-firing laser catheters met with only limited success. This was principally due to the inability of the urologists to direct laser energy laterally into obstructing prostatic lobes to achieve maximum ablation. The development of side-firing or right-angled delivery systems has revolutionized laser treatment of benign prostatic hyperplasia (BPH).

It was not until the advent of laser treatment of BPH that lasers became universally accepted as part of the urological armamentarium. The Nd:YAG laser has been used to treat superficial papillary bladder tumours without conferring a significant advantage over conventional electrocautery resection of bladder carcinoma. The Tunable dye laser has been used to obliterate stones in the ureter, but owing to the high cost of the Tunable dye machines there has been little universal enthusiasm for this form of laser technology in a benign condition. Lasers have also been used to treat superficial penile carcinoma, allowing precise excision of lesions with a good cosmetic and functional result, possibly sparing partial penectomy for some patients. Another burgeoning area of theoretical laser application in benign conditions is the use of the laser in tissue welding. There have been mainly experimental animal reports of Nd:YAG, carbon dioxide (CO_2), argon and diode laser wavelengths to produce sutureless tissue fusion. The majority of these reports have been in the animal experimental model. Vasovasostomy and artificially fashioned hypospadias in the rat model have been repaired using a sutureless tissue fusion with various laser wave-lengths.[1] There have been several reports in the literature of laser-assisted vasectomy reversal using a combination of suture and laser thermal energy to form a tissue fusion. More recently, the addition of fibrin glue and laser thermal energy has improved tissue fusion and has made it more likely that clinical application in vasectomy reversal will occur.

However, it has been in the area of BPH that the laser is having its most significant impact in urological surgery. For 60 years, since first described by Nesbitt,[2] transurethral resection of the prostate (TURP) has been the predominant urological operation, occupying 38% of the urologist's workload. Although TURP produces an excellent patient outcome in 80% of patients, approximately 20% of patients express some dissatisfaction with this procedure.[3] A surprisingly high incidence of morbidity, bleeding, hyponatraemia, infection, incontinence and blood transfusion, and a 16–20% reoperation rate at 5 years, have prompted a more critical appraisal of this stock procedure. The operative technique of TURP is difficult to learn and requires several years of supervised tuition by a skilled resectionist. Because an irrigating bladder catheter is normally required to evacuate blood clots postoperatively, patients remain in hospital for 2–5 days following surgery. This makes the procedure costly with regard to the length of hospital stay. Morbidity, combined with the high cost of TURP, has led to the evaluation of transurethral microwave thermal therapy, focused ultrasound, intraurethral balloon dilatation and intraurethral coils and springs, and medication to reduce prostatic volume, as less morbid alternatives to TURP. However, these techniques have not delivered clinically measured outcome parameters equivalent to those with TURP. The use of the side-firing laser to treat obstructing prostatic adenoma was first described in 1990, at St Vincent's Hospital in Melbourne. The first patient treatment was in October 1990.[4]

Previously, Roth and Aretz[5] first demonstrated the potential of laser-induced prostatectomy in the canine model. Initial reports from Roth described a transurethral ultrasound-guided laser-induced prostatectomy (TULIP) procedure. This canine feasibility study demonstrated the efficacy of high-power laser ablation of the prostate, reflecting the laser beam at right angles into the prostate under ultrasound guidance.

Johnson and associates[6] reported that a right-angled delivery fibre introduced through standard endoscope equipment transurethrally could produce similar results under direct visual application of laser light. Johnson's canine studies paved the way for the clinical application of laser thermal energy in human BPH.

Johnson used a 600 μm quartz light guide attached to a Nd:YAG generator. The quartz light guide had a stainless steel reflecting dish coated with gold glued to its tip. Light was brought through the dish and reflected at 90 degrees from a highly polished gold mirror. This laser catheter had been used in the treatment of human endometrial disease to cause endometrial ablation. Early dosimetry studies,[4] using a variety of power settings both in the canine and potato model, suggested that a 60 W power setting for 60 s would produce the deepest zone of coagulative necrosis in the prostate. Subsequent authors—Kabalin[7] and Cammach and colleagues[8]—have suggested that lower power settings used for a longer lasing time will produce equivalent or improved coagulative necrosis. Appropriate dosimetry has yet to be defined finally in the treatment of human prostatic adenoma disease.

Fibre technology

Subsequent to earlier reports of the TULIP method and the gold-plated side-firing catheters, prism-type angled-beam delivery systems have been developed. The Ultraline® catheter from Heraeus is a glass prism with internal refraction delivering energy to the adenoma. The Prolase II catheter also uses an internal prism refrating-type technology. These catheters do allow more tissue contact and produce more surface vaporization than the free-beam angled delivery devices. Recently, Daughtry and Rodan[9] have demonstrated the feasibility of using an enlarged sapphire contact tip to perform contact laser TURP. Johnson et al[10] have also recently reported the use of interstitial thermal therapy (ITT) to produce a gross and histopathologically confirmed interstitial laser prostatectomy in the canine model. This model demonstrated distinct zonal thermal changes surrounding the entire active area of the ITT fibre. A large well-demarcated area of acute coagulative necrosis occurred immediately surrounding each fibre tract. Beyond this were prominent narrow peripheral zones of marked tissue disruption and an outer zone of haemorrhage. Liquefaction within these coagulative areas was evident in 24 h and by 4 days each lobe of the prostate contained an irregular cavity that became lined by normal-appearing transitional epithelium. By 5 weeks this communicated with the prostatic urethra. These canine studies by Johnson on ITT have been validated by Muschter et al,[11] who reported ITT in 350 human clinical studies with an outcome equivalent to that with conventional TURP. Muschter's technique has the advantage of leaving the urethra intact while causing an internal coagulative necrosis. The necrotic tissue of the prostate is not sloughed but absorbed, leaving atrophy and scar formation. The shrinking process requires 4–12 weeks but does not seem to be accompanied by some of the irritative symptoms associated with the free-beam technology. Muschter used a Nd:YAG laser in combination with specially designed light guides (600 μm quartz glass fibre with diffuser tip, 2 cm in length and 1.9 mm in diameter).

Recently Muschter[12] has also used a diode laser (830 nm) with special application-type fibres. In the interstitial technique, the tip of the light guide is inserted into the bulky prostatic adenoma transurethrally through a cystoscope and fibre placement numbers depend on the size and configuration of the prostate. As many as 15 interstitial treatments can be given. In interstitial laser therapy the laser can be used at much lower power settings than in the free-beam technique, and a power setting of 5–7 W appears to suffice.

The first study of successful patient treatments with side-firing gold mirror laser catheters that demonstrated safety and efficacy was published in 1992[13] (Fig. 21.1). Seventeen patients with bladder neck obstruction due to BPH were treated with a Nd:YAG laser with a 60 W power setting. Initially, a prototype deflecting gold-alloy tip on a quartz laser fibre (Lateralase) was used. This initial report describes the simple, rapid and bloodless technique of laser prostatectomy. However, the authors were guarded in the conclusion that this was universally applicable. In an initial pilot study,[4] four patients were treated at 60 W continuous wave for 1 min in four quadrants, treating the roof of the prostatic fossa and the floor as well as both lateral lobes. A 4 min lasing time was used in this technique and the laser was directed posteriorly towards the rectum. This had been the technique developed by Johnson et al[6] in canine studies and very low joule numbers were used to treat the prostatic adenoma. The median lobe was treated separately with a short burst of laser energy for less than 1 min. Using this technique it was possible to treat patients with prostatic volumes up to 30 cm^3 only; it was difficult to achieve adequate vaporization and cavitation in prostates larger than this volume with this dosimetry regimen. In patients with prostates greater than 30 cm^3 in volume, where the posterior urethral length exceeded 3 cm, a significant residue of obstructing lateral lobe adenoma persisted. The intense heat generated in this prototype gold-alloy reflector often caused the tip to melt after lasing for 3–4 min, particularly if the tip came into contact with prostatic tissue. In

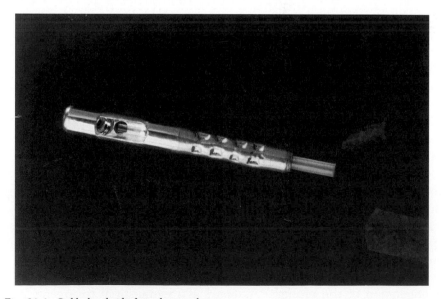

Fig. 21.1. Gold-plated side-firing laser catheter.

several of the patients studied, laser time was considerably less than 4 min because of meltdown of the tip. However, there was no significant bleeding and patient outcome appeared satisfactory. In the development of this technique it was clearly necessary for the fibre tip to be stationed above the verumontanum to protect the external urethral sphincter, since inadvertent lasing of the external sphincter could cause significant sphincter damage or complete destruction, with subsequent incontinence. However, no patient in this study became incontinent.

Patients were initially returned to the ward without an indwelling catheter; however, it became apparent that the burning and tissue oedema at the bladder neck and in the posterior urethra following laser at a high-power setting of 60 W caused voiding difficulty and 50% of these patients went into urinary retention. The catheter was therefore placed in the urethra for 2–3 days while the oedema subsided. However a non-irrigating catheter was all that was necessary, as no bleeding occurred and clot retention was not a problem.

An average of 1800 kJ was used per patient, with a mean lasing time of 4.2 min. Symptom scores in this group of 17 patients fell from a mean of 15 preoperatively to a mean of 4 at 6 weeks and preoperative flow rate rose from a mean of 5 ml to a postoperative rate of 9 ml/s at 6 weeks (Table 21.1). Thus, only a modest improvement in flow rate was seen. Flexible urethroscope under local anaesthesia revealed the presence of residual occlusive tissue in seven patients at 6 weeks following laser therapy. This study demonstrated that the procedure was safe, even when the laser beam was directed at 6 o'clock in the posterior urethra directly towards the rectum: there was no suggestion of rectal heating or rectal damage using this technique. It was also clear that the 6 week evaluation was too early and that significant tissue slough was likely to occur following the 6 week interval, unlike the situation in canine studies where there is almost immediate cavitation following laser therapy in the dog prostate. This pilot study demonstrated feasibility of laser prostatectomy but certainly did not demonstrate clinical efficacy equivalent to that with conventional TURP. It also demonstrated that the results of canine studies could not be

Parameter*	Assessment			
	Preoperative		Postoperative (6 weeks)	
	Mean	Range	Mean	Range
AUA symptom score	15	8–21	4	1–10
Q_{max} (ml/s)	5	0–15	9	0–21

Table 21.1. Results of a pilot study of 17 patients treated by laser ablation of the prostate
*AUA, American Urological Association; Q_{max}, peak urinary flow rate.

extrapolated to the human prostate. This first study using side-firing technology followed the work of McPhee[14] in 1989 using a Nd:YAG laser after TURP to improve haemostasis. However, this technique was cumbersome and there was some difficulty in controlling bleeding from large vessels of the bladder neck. Beisland and Stranden[15] in 1984 used Nd:YAG laser energy 3–4 weeks after TURP to treat localized prostate cancer but found it necessary to insert the flexible laser cable into the prostatic cavity through a suprapubic trocar cystoscope. The procedure was well tolerated and devoid of serious complications, and preliminary results were encouraging. Similarly, McNicholas[16] in 1990 used the Nd:YAG laser after an extended TURP to treat early carcinoma of the prostate, with no immediate alteration in continence or potency.

Second-generation delivery systems for laser prostatic ablation

Improvements in fibre technology subsequently occurred. A refined side-firing laser catheter was developed by the Myriadlase® Corporation (Arlington, TX, USA). This device was a refinement of the original prototype Lateralase system. The device comprised a solid gold tip of 99% purity incorporating a flat mirror that deflected the central ray of the beam emerging from the flat end of the 600 μm diameter fibre through a 105 degree angle, resulting in a laterally directed beam. Gold was chosen as the material comprising the entire tip primarily because of its high index of reflectivity of more than 98% for a wavelength greater than 1 μm (which includes the 1.064 μm (1064 nm) wavelength of the surgical Nd:YAG laser), its high thermal conductivity (3.15 W/cm^2), and its relative inertness to body tissue and fluids (biocompatability). The monolithic design of pure gold was chosen to optimize both volume heat transfer and heat sinking to the aqueous irrigating solution normally used during laser coagulation of tissue. The lack of surface oxidation and relative resistance to build-up of proteinaceous material on the surface of the gold tip serves to maintain heat sinking during lasing in irrigated body cavities at Nd:YAG laser input power up to 80 W. This fibre tip also contained a venturi hole which minimized the adherence of debris to the fibre tip and prevented a build-up of proteinaceous material on the mirror, which can ruin its reflectivity. The device was attached to a 600 μm light guide.

Thirty-three men were treated using this new side-fibre durable laser catheter.[17] In this pilot study a power setting of 60 W was used. The technique of lasing in the posterior urethra was changed to avoid direct posterior lasing; similarly the roof of the prostate was not lased at 12 o'clock. In a technique described by Cowles,[18] lasing of the lateral lobes was delivered in four quadrants in a circumferential fashion at the 2, 4, 8 and 10 o'clock positions (Fig. 21.2). Lasing was for 1 min continuously at 60 W, with slow water irrigation through a 23 Fr cystoscope using a 30 degree telescope. The catheter was kept above the verumontanum at all times to prevent inadvertent sphincter damage. The median lobe was lased after a satisfactory lateral lobe ablation and a power setting of 60 W for 60 s was also used. If the urethral length was more than 3–3.5 cm, indicating a larger prostate, a second circumferential lasing was performed, closer to the bladder neck. In some cases a third circumferential lasing was performed. Thus, increasing doses of laser energy were used in this study. A mean dose of 25 677 J was used, with a maximum dose of 54 390 J in one patient. Epidural anaesthesia was used in most cases, with general anaesthesia being used in two cases in this study where patients received anticoagulants during treatment.

The American Urological Association (AUA) symptom score fell from a preoperative mean of 21.47 to 9.5 postoperatively and flow rate increased from a Q_{max} of 8.5 ml/s to 15.24 ml/s (Table 21.2). Thus the authors, by increasing the dose of laser energy used and specifically targetting obstructing adenoma in the lateral lobes, were able to achieve a clinically unobstructed flow rate at the 3 month interval. Again, in this study bleeding was not a problem, with no blood transfusions and no postoperative clot retention, even in the patients on full anticoagulant therapy. This newer fibre system appeared to be more durable and the

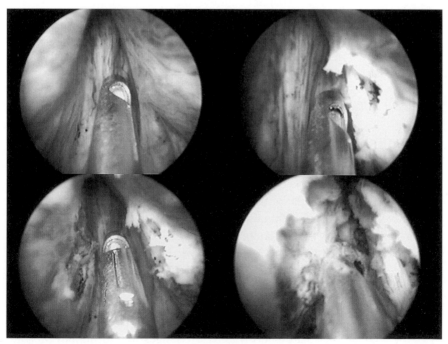

Fig. 21.2. Four-quadrant lasing.

Parameter*	Assessment			
	Preoperative		Postoperative (3 months)	
	Mean	Range	Mean	Range
AUA symptom score	21.47	8–35	9.5	0–20
Q_{max} (ml/s)	8.5	3.1–16.6	15.24	6.8–32.7
Q_{ave} (ml/s)	4.35	1.5–8.4	7.7	2.7–15.8
PVR (ml)	109.5	11–620	48	13–172

Table 21.2. Second-generation technology: clinical outcome of laser ablation of the prostate in 33 patients

*AUA, American Urological Association; Q_{max}, Q_{ave}, peak and average urinary flow rates; PVR, post-voiding residual.

addition of the venturi aperture on this side-fire catheter seemed to preserve it from overheating, distortion and destruction following tissue adherence. In earlier studies, fibre disintegration often occurred before 4 min lasing. Mean lasing time rose from 4.2 min to 6.8 min in this study. Modification of the laser ablation technique, which avoided lasing at the 6 and 12 o'clock positions, enabled lateral lobe destruction to be increased; this was confirmed cystoscopically. However, the authors noted that there seemed to be some variability of ablation effect from patient to patient, independent of prostatic volume. There may be variability in prostatic optical density in individual prostates, causing a variation in tissue effect. This may be due to a variation in stromal epithelial ratios in each prostate, causing a difference in forward scatter of the laser light at the 1064 nm wavelength. Concerns regarding this therapy remained, related to fibre cost, absence of evaluable tissue for histological examination and the prolonged urinary retention in some patients.

Histopathological changes in human prostatic adenoma following Nd:YAG laser ablation therapy

Removal of prostatic tissue by endoscopic resection or open surgical techniques from seven patients who had previously undergone attempted prostatic laser ablation therapy offered an opportunity to evaluate sequential effects of such energy on the human prostate at varying intervals after treatment.[19] A progressive inflammatory and necrotic response initially akin to that demonstrated following a thermal burn, together with evolving vascular changes within residual viable prostate tissue, are demonstrated. Six patients who underwent TURP and one radical prostatectomy at intervals after visual laser ablation of the prostate (VLAP) were studied to demonstrate the changes in the human prostate whereby Nd:YAG laser energy causes a deep coagulative necrosis and arterial thrombosis in prostatic adenoma. These changes, however, differed significantly from those seen in reported canine studies.[5,6] A slower cavitation effect is seen in the human compared with the canine, mirroring the continuing clinical effect in voiding parameters over time. Canine cavitation after laser energy delivery occurs almost completely by 4–6 weeks, whereas in humans residual tissue slough can be seen as long as 10 months following lasing. In human prostatic adenoma, a marked acute inflammation with haemorrhagic necrosis occurs after lasing and this is followed by chronic changes of ischaemic necrosis developing months after treatment. All patients were treated with 60 W for 60 s.

Results

All specimens showed a considerable tissue effect after laser treatment. These changes in the histological appearance of the resected tissue varied with the duration of time after lasing, showing a gradual and progressive response. In a prostate resected immediately following transurethral laser therapy, evidence of cellular damage akin to that closely following upon a thermal burn was identified. This consisted of cellular disruption with surrounding oedema and signs of early inflammatory cell infiltrate. These features were distinct from the appearance of the prostate gland of the same patient in a transrectal biopsy taken 1 week before surgery, which demonstrated only uncomplicated BPH together with a mild lymphocyte and macrophage infiltrate thought to represent mild chronic prostatitis. The acute prostatic changes consequent upon laser energy in this resection specimen were also thought to be only superficial in distribution, with the visible tissue effects usually not being present across the complete width of affected prostatic chips, and with the majority of the resected tissue appearing to be unaffected by the laser energy.

More extensive tissue damage was identified in the specimen obtained at transurethral resection 7 days following laser ablation of the prostate gland. Greater distribution of necrotic tissue was evident than in the earlier specimen and there was evidence of a neutrophil infiltration and significant haemorrhage into the denatured tissue in the zone of necrosis. Areas of preserved nuclear architecture with apparent nuclear viability, as determined by staining of DNA with haematoxylin, were also present within the region of necrosis. A transition zone with some chips from necrotic to viable tissue could also be identified, although the depth of this differentiation within the prostate gland could not be determined. In the sections of viable prostatic tissue immediately adjacent to the necrotic region, a marked inflammatory cell infiltrate was present. Also present in this specimen were prominent vascular thromboses with fibrin staining evident within vessels. Such signs of vascular occlusion were present extensively within the zone of tissue necrosis but were additionally identified in bundles within the prostatic tissue well peripheral to the region of demarcation of viable adenoma. This histological feature was common to almost all of the later resection specimens following transurethral laser ablation of the prostate, with these changes in vascular perfusion extending significantly peripheral to the inner limit of tissue viability. The specimen from the patient who underwent radical prostatectomy 28 days after laser therapy was subjected to a detailed macroscopic and microscopic examination. Macroscopic inspection revealed a 1.5 cm diameter cuff of white necrotic tissue around the prostatic urethra with a more peripheral haemorrhagic and erythematous zone surrounding it. The total diameter of these areas of altered prostatic tissue was 2.7 cm. Histological examination again confirmed that the central white zone represented coagulative necrosis with complete loss of cell detail, and that the peripheral region showed extensive haemorrhage into regions of additional coagulative necrosis and granulation tissue formation, as had been seen in earlier resected specimens. However, distinct evidence of recanalization of blood vessels was now present at the interface between necrotic and viable tissue more centrally than had previously been observed. Subsequent resected specimens between 37 days and 10 months demonstrated significant vascular changes. Early changes in response to injury and infarction appeared to evolve to produce a squamous change in glandular epithelium, with many cells displaying keratinization with opaque cytoplasm; there was also extensive fibrosis. In addition, those vessels visible within the resected specimen demonstrated numerous abnormal histological characteristics, particularly when identified at the margin of the necrotic zone. Arteries appeared thick-walled and telangiectatic, with abnormal muscles within their walls, displaying features somewhat similar to those identified several months after radiotherapy-induced vascular damage.

It appears that the improvements in flow rate and symptom score after laser therapy are the results of a progressive denaturation of prostatic tissue, with such altered adenoma probably constituting the tissue slough that is passed in the urine by patients after treatment.

The histological changes demonstrated within the prostate gland at various intervals after treatment are similar in nature to those reported previously after microwave hyperthermia. Tissue damage appears to result from a thermal burn to the prostate gland in the initial phase of treatment. The presence of prominent vascular thrombosis, both within necrotic tissue and in viable adenoma peripherally, invites speculation on the contribution and ongoing role of ischaemia with regard to the later changes seen following transurethral application of laser energy. Evidence of necrotic tissue in the resection specimen at 10 months after treatment, together with identification of extensive squamous change and keratinization in residual adenomatous tissue, is more consistent with such an aetiology than the result of a purely thermal energy. There appears to be a combination of thermal damage causing coagulative necrosis, and late vascular thrombosis. This vascular thrombosis causes ischaemia of the transition zone of the prostate. Such transition zone infarction may explain the continued satisfactory clinical outcome in patients 12–24 months following laser therapy. This study[19] is in contrast to studies in which laser treatment was administered to the canine prostate, where 50% of the necrotic tissue was sloughed within 5 days of therapy and complete re-epithelialization of the urethra had taken place by 3 weeks.[6]

Such conflicting results between the human and canine model may be accounted for in part by the substantially lower stromal:epithelial ratio seen in the canine prostate when compared with the human analogue. It may be that prostatic adenoma of the composition more typical of the canine prostate model has greater sensitivity to the effects of thermal energy than human adenoma, in which a higher stromal content is evident.

Caution should therefore be exercised when attempts are made to correlate canine and human studies. In the canine there is a substantial difference in laser tissue effect at various power settings. Cystic cavitation seen in the canine at 4 weeks did not occur in the human until much later. There was no clinical evidence of capsular penetration, periprostatic or rectal effect of laser energy at a 60 W power setting in the treatment of human prostatic adenoma.

Phase III studies of laser prostatectomy

Since the original reports[4,13] of the efficacy and safety of laser prostatectomy, a phase III report from Dixon et al[20] has been published, demonstrating excellent clinical outcome equivalent to that which could be expected from TURP following laser prostatectomy. A randomized study[21] comparing TURP with VLAP in 71 patients has shown equivalent outcome in the measurable clinical parameters Q_{max} increase and AUA symptom score reduction at 6 months (Tables 21.3 and 21.4). Another study[22] of 22 men on full anticoagulant therapy, treated with laser prostatectomy without withdrawal of anticoagulants, suggests that there may be a clear advantage in this cohort of patients in the choice of laser over conventional electrocautery resection. The ability of the urologist to treat patients on anticoagulant therapy without withdrawing the anti-coagulation and without risk of bleeding makes laser treatment very useful in this patient group.

Costello[23] has reported a case of successful treatment of an HIV-positive male in acute retention treated by VLAP. These HIV-positive patients constitute a risk to operating personnel and operating-room staff and ward personnel. Concern over the risk of virus transmission from irrigant

Assessment	VLAP			TURP			Significance
	n	Mean (SD)	Range	n	Mean (SD)	Range	
Preop	34	19.94 (7.6)	9–35	37	20.97 (5.9)	6–35	NS $p=0.52$
6 weeks	32	13.73 (6.5)	0–24	37	7.76 (5.4)	0–22	$p=0.001$
3 months	30	10.5 (5.6)	0–21	29	6 (4.1)	0–15	$p=0.002$
6 months	25	9.27 (7.4)	0–30	25	4.43 (4.4)	0–16	$p=0.01$

Table 21.3. Clinical outcome at 6 months: AUA symptom score after visual laser ablation of the prostate (VLAP) vs transurethral resection of the prostate (TURP)

Assessment	VLAP			TURP			Significance
	n	Mean (SD)	Range	n	Mean (SD)	Range	
Preop	34	8.76 (3.6)	3–15	37	9.48 (3.6)	3.2–17.3	NS $p=0.42$
6 weeks	32	12.79 (6.6)	3.2–37.1	37	16.44 (5.5)	6.6–27.2	$p=0.02$
3 months	30	14.35 (6.3)	3.7–33	29	17.83 (8.1)	6.6–43.6	NS $p=0.09$
6 months	25	15.74 (9.1)	4.9–31	25	19.1 (12.1)	4.4–53.6	NS $p=0.35$

Table 21.4. Clinical outcome at 6 months: peak urine flow rates (ml/s) after VLAP vs TURP

splash and postoperative irrigation following TURP is quite considerable. The almost complete bloodlessness of the laser procedure, compared with conventional electrocautery, makes it a procedure of choice in this patient group.

Anaesthesia for laser prostatectomy

A study by Costello and Costello[24] suggests that epidural anaesthesia may be the preferred anaesthesia type for laser prostatectomy. In this study of 72 patients undergoing laser TURP, the most serious complication of conventional TURP (that of blood transfusion) was obviated; in addition, there was no evidence of the syndrome of water intoxication. The laser procedure is essentially bloodless as no prostatic venous sinuses are opened. The laser light penetrates deeply into tissue, causing immediate thrombosis and coagulative necrosis. The lack of clots in the bladder, due to absence of prostatic cavity bleeding, obviates the requirement for continuous postoperative bladder irrigation, thus further reducing the possibility of water intoxication. Theatre and ward staff are not exposed to the combined hazards of contact with blood-stained irrigant fluid and to administration of blood transfusion, with the attendant risk of virus transmission to staff. Laser TURP offers a major advance in the management of medically unfit patients. The average lasing time is short, 15 min on average. The absence of blood transfusion, fluid shift and electrolyte disturbance provides the anaesthetist with a safer anaesthetic environment for the management of the elderly and physically severely compromised BPH patient. The use of short-duration local anaesthetic agents as part of the epidural technique in this series allows for early ambulation. Because of this, laser TURP seems increasingly appropriate to the outpatient setting. Regional anaesthesia by either the epidural or the spinal route would seem ideal for the patient undergoing laser TURP. Measurements of serum sodium, serum potassium and free haemoglobin immediately after surgery and 24 h after laser prostatectomy demonstrate no statistically different level between pre- and postoperative readings. Leach et al[25] have reported local anaesthesia in laser prostatectomy in 46 patients, with good outcome.

Nursing and laser ablation of the prostate

Following conventional TURP, specialized nursing skills are required to keep the urinary catheter patent in the presence of postoperative bleeding.[26] Maintenance of continuous bladder irrigation, observation of urinary flow and prompt attention to clot retention with manual bladder washouts, when necessary, are time-consuming labour-intensive nursing activities. The patient's mobility and independence are limited by bladder irrigation; this also increases demands for nursing assistance. Following laser prostatectomy, as there is no significant bleeding and no irrigation or bladder washout, nursing activities are much less than for TURP patients. Studies that compared patient–nurse dependency ratios and nursing-hour requirements of laser prostatectomy and TURP have demonstrated a reduced requirement for nuring after laser prostatectomy. Another benefit of the bloodlessness of laser prostatectomy is the shorter bed stay, as patients are not required to remain in hospital beyond initial postsurgical recovery, and can return home on the same day. Shorter bed stay and the need to ensure that the patients have realistic expectations of their surgical outcome following laser prostatectomy means that there is a necessity for nurses to provide appropriate preoperative and perioperative education. Patients may have unrealistic expectations of laser surgery and this should be fully discussed and modified before surgery. Patients should be aware of the plan to discharge them home with the catheter in situ, and should be given instructions for management of their catheter and leg bag at home. Most important is the education regarding postoperative irritative symptoms, which can last for up to 6 weeks following laser prostatectomy. There is also a small risk of urinary retention following laser prostatectomy after catheter removal at 5 days and patients should be aware of this. Some patients will require antispasmodics to treat the urgency and frequency, and this should be explained before surgery. In hospitals where laser prostatectomy is currently being performed there has been a shift in nursing emphasis, from the specialized clinical skills required to care for a patient with post-prostatectomy bleeding to the educational skills needed to ensure that these patients are informed about, and prepared for, the outcome of their surgery.

Conclusions

In the 4 years since the first clinical descriptions of laser prostatectomy this operation has now come to challenge the predominant TURP as an appropriate surgical option for treatment of BPH. The advent of cheaper, more durable laser delivery systems will speed up the acceptance of the technique. It remains to be seen whether other laser wavelengths, such as the diode wavelength between 800 and 900 nm or the holmium wavelength at 2040 nm, will improve laser prostatectomy. It appears that technical refinements and increased familiarity with laser surgery by urologists will ensure the lasting role of laser prostatectomy in urological surgery.

References

1. Shanberg A, Tansey L, Baghdassaruan K et al. Laser assisted vasectomy reversal: experience in 32 patients. J Urol 1990; 143: 528–530
2. Nesbitt R M. Transurethral prostatectomy. Baltimore: Charles C. Thomas, 1943
3. Doll H A, Black N A, McPherson K et al. Mortality, morbidity and complications following transurethral resection of the prostate for benign prostatic hypertrophy. J Urol 1992; 147: 1566–1573
4. Costello A J, Johnson D E, Bolton D M. Nd:YAG laser ablation of the prostate as a treatment for benign prostatic hypertrophy. Lasers Surg Med 1992; 12: 121–124
5. Roth R, Aretz H. Transurethral ultrasound guided laser induced prostatectomy (TULIP procedure): a canine prostate feasibility study. J Urol 1991; 146: 1128–1135
6. Johnson D E, Levinson A K, Greskovitch F J et al. Transurethral laser prostatectomy using a right-angle laser delivery system. SPIE Proc 1991; 1421: 36–41
7. Kabalin J N. Laser prostatectomy performed with a right angle firing neodymium:YAG laser fibre at 40 watts power setting. J Urol 1993; 150: 95
8. Cammach J T, Motamedi M, Torres J H et al. Endoscopic Nd:YAG laser coagulation of the prostate: comparison of low power versus high power. J Urol 1993; 149: 4, 215A (abstr 5)
9. Daughtry J D, Rodan B A. Transurethral laser prostatectomy: a comparison of contact tip mode and lateral firing free beam mode. J Clin Laser Med Surg 1993; 11: 21–27

10. Johnson D E, Cromeens D M, Price R E. Interstitial laser prostatectomy. Lasers Surg Med 1994; 14: 299–305
11. Muschter R, Hessel S, Hofstetter A et al. One year experience in interstitial laser coagulation for benign prostatic hyperplasia. J Urol 1993; 149: 466 (abstr)
12. Muschter R. Personal communication, 1994
13. Costello A J, Bowsher W G, Bolton D M et al. Laser ablation of the prostate in patients with benign prostatic hypertrophy. Br J Urol 1992; 69: 603–605
14. McPhee M S. Lasers in urologic surgery, 2nd ed. Chicago: Year Book Medical, 1989: 41–49
15. Beisland H O, Stranden E. Rectal temperature monitoring during neodymium:YAG laser irradiation for prostatic carcinoma. Urol Res 1984; 12: 257–259
16. McNicholas T A. Lasers in urology in principle and practice. London: Springer-Verlag, 1990: 63–82
17. Costello A J, Shaffer B S, Crowe H R. Second-generation delivery systems for laser prostatic ablation. Urology 1994; 43: 262–266
18. Cowles R S, III. Visual laser ablation of the prostate. In: Cooner W H (ed) Mediguide to urology. New York: Delacorte, 1993; 1–4
19. Costello A J, Bolton D M, Ellis D, Crowe H. Histopathological changes in human prostatic adenoma following Nd:YAG laser ablation therapy. J Urol 1994; 152: 1526–1529
20. Dixon C, Machi G, Theven C, Lepor H. A prospective, double-blind, randomized study comparing laser ablation of the prostate and transurethral prostatectomy for the treatment of BPH. J Urol 1993; 149: 215A (abstr)
21. Costello A J, Crowe H R, Jackson T, Street A. A randomized single institution study comparing laser prostatectomy and transurethral resection of the prostate. Ann Acad Med Singapore 1994; in press
22. Kingston T E, Nonnenmacher A K, Crowe H et al. Further evaluation of transurethral laser ablation of the prostate in patients treated with anticoagulant therapy. Aust NZ J Surg 1994; in press
23. Costello A J. Laser prostatectomy in an HIV positive male. Aust Med J 1993; 159: 286
24. Costello T J, Costello A J. Anaesthesia for laser prostatectomy. Anaesth Intensive Care 1994; 22: 454–457
25. Leach G E, Sirls L, Ganabathi K et al. Outpatient visual laser assisted prostatectomy under local anaesthesia. Urology 1994; 43: 149–153
26. Crowe H R, Costello A J. Laser ablation of the prostate: nursing management. Urol Nurs 1994; 14: 38–40

Percutaneous cryosurgery for the management of advanced renal cell carcinoma

22

M. Uchida   K. Yoneda   H. Watanabe

Introduction

The main treatment for renal cell carcinoma is radical nephrectomy. However, patients with advanced renal cell carcinoma involving severe macrohaematuria are difficult to treat because chemotherapy, the administration of interferon and embolization from the renal artery are not sufficiently effective.

Recently, the percutaneous technique with interventional ultrasound has made rapid progress in urology as a minimally invasive form of surgery. The fundamental studies and clinical application as a new modality for advanced renal cell carcinoma by a combination of the percutaneous technique and cryotherapy are described in this chapter.

Development of a probe for percutaneous cryosurgery

An original cryoprobe was developed for the purpose. The probe was 6.8 mm in diameter, and the tip was 30 mm in length (Fig. 22.1). The probe was attached to a Spembly cryosurgical system 130, which employs liquid nitrogen for freezing.

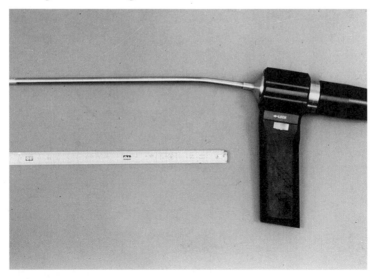

Fig. 22.1. Original probe (6.8 mm in diameter) for percutaneous cryosurgery.

An ice ball 30 mm in diameter developed around the tip of the probe during a cooling time of 5 min in a water tank kept at 40°C. The cooling function of the probe was similar to that of a conventional probe.

Tolerance test of renal cell cancer cells by cooling

No reports have been available on the sensitivity of renal cell cancer cells to cooling. In order to examine the tolerance of renal cell cancer cells to cooling, renal cell cancer cell lines (NC-65) were frozen under sterile conditions in an ultralow freezer for 60 min at temperatures of −5, −10, −20 and −30°C. Renal cell cancer cell viability was calculated at each temperature after 24 h with a phase contrast microscope.

Although 95–96% of renal cell cancer cells survived after cooling for 60 min above −10°C only 15% survived below −20°C (Fig. 22.2). In

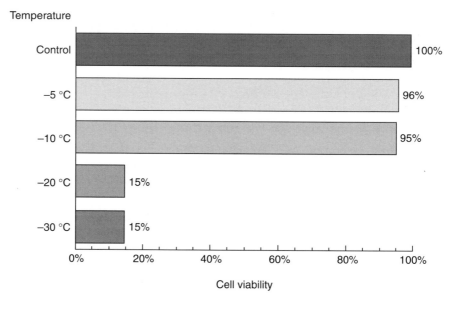

Fig. 22.2. Renal cell cancer cell viability at temperatures of −5 to −30°C.

renal cell cancer cells cooled below −20°C, the border of the cytoplasm was indistinct and the nucleoli disappeared. The results suggested that a temperature below −20°C is required for the cryonecrosis of renal cell cancer cells.

Cooling test of human kidneys with renal cell cancer

The kidney is a deeply situated organ with an internal blood flow of 400–500 ml/min. Cryosurgery of such organs has, therefore, not usually been contemplated. Cooling tests of two nephrectomized kidneys with hypervascular renal cell cancer, approximately 50 mm in size, were performed in water at 40°C. The cryoprobe was inserted into the centre of the tumour. Thermometers 1 mm in diameter were placed 1 and 2 cm away from the probe. After nephrectomy, heparin sodium was injected from the renal artery to prevent coagulation. One kidney was irrigated with saline at 40°C from the renal artery at a rate of 400 ml/min, while the other kidney was not irrigated. The condition of the specimen with irrigation simulated the kidney in vivo and that without irrigation simulated the kidney after embolization.

An ice ball formed in the tumour 30 min after cooling, with or without irrigation. The temperature in the tumour without irrigation fell rapidly 5 min later and stabilized 15 min later at $-75°C$ in the region 1 cm from the probe and at $-45°C$ in the region 2 cm from the probe. The temperature in the tumour with irrigation fell slowly and was stabilized 30 min later at $-12°C$ in the area 1 cm from the probe and at $-8°C$ in the area 2 cm away. The results suggested that in order to treat hypervascular renal cell cancers, embolization of the renal artery may be necessary as a pretreatment.

Influence of cryosurgery on the normal tissue in the kidney

To assess the influence of cryosurgery on the normal tissue in the kidney, the right kidneys of two dogs were exposed under ketamine anaesthesia. The cryoprobe was inserted into the middle of each kidney from the lower pole and cooling was performed for 2 min. After cooling, the abdomen was closed. The kidney was examined macroscopically and microscopically 1 week after cooling (short follow-up) in one dog and 12 weeks after cooling (long follow-up) in the other.

In both dogs the whole kidney was frozen in 2 min. In the short follow-up case, a wedge-shaped portion with haematoma following the route of the probe was observed macroscopically. The frozen kidney was almost equal to the other kidney in size (Fig. 22.3a). No adhesions were seen between the frozen kidney and the surrounding organs. Infiltration of erythrocytes and lymphocytes in both the cortex and medulla of the wedge-shaped portion was seen microscopically (Fig. 22.3b). In the long follow-up case, the frozen kidney was smaller than the other kidney (Fig. 22.4a). Microscopic examination of the frozen kidney showed an atrophic change with scarring, as well as shrunken glomeruli (Fig. 22.4b). This meant that cryosurgery had the effect of autonephrectomy.

Clinical application of percutaneous cryosurgery for advanced renal cell carcinoma

Three patients with advanced renal cell cancer were selected for the

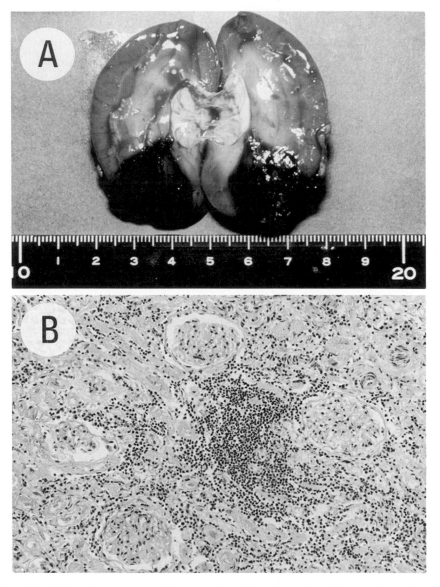

Fig. 22.3. Effect of cryosurgery on the normal dog kidney after a short follow-up (1 week after cooling): (A) macroscopic findings; (B) microscopic findings. (Haematoxylin and eosin, reduced from × 200.)

clinical application of percutaneous cryosurgery. Patient 1 was a 48-year-old male with complaints of vesical tamponade due to macrohaematuria and dyspnoea. Urological examination revealed a left renal cell carcinoma with para-aortic lymph node swelling and lymphangitis carcinomatosis. Respiratory assistance was needed. Patient 2, a 65-year-old male, complained of macrohaematuria and severe pain in the pelvic bone. Urological examination revealed a right renal cell carcinoma with

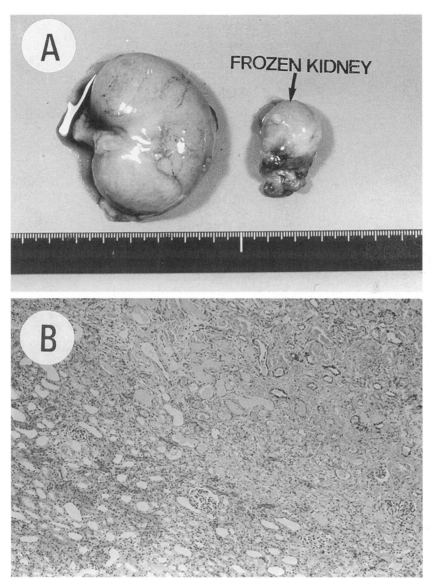

Fig. 22.4. Effect of cryosurgery on the normal dog kidney after a long follow-up (12 weeks after cooling): (A) macroscopic findings; (B) microscopic findings. (Haematoxylin and eosin, reduced from ×100.)

metastases to the lung and the pelvic bone. Epidural anaesthesia was required. Patient 3, a 62-year-old male, complained of general fatigue, a severe cough and loss of body weight. Urological examination revealed a right renal cell carcinoma with multiple lung metastases and tumour thrombus to the inferior vena cava. In all patients, embolization of the renal artery and the administration of interferon were performed initially, but the disease was progressive. The Karnofsky performance scales were 10,

40 and 60%, respectively, for the three patients. Informed consent was obtained for percutaneous cryosurgery.

The patients were placed on a surgical table in the prone position under general anaesthesia. Percutaneous puncture with interventional ultrasound using an 18 G needle was performed at the centre of the renal tumour. A guide wire was inserted into the tumour and the puncture tract was dilated to 24 Fr. A sheath of 24 Fr made of Teflon to prevent heat conductivity was put in place and the cryoprobe was inserted through the sheath. At the same time, two thermometers 0.5 mm in diameter were placed 1 cm from the probe inside the tumour and the margin between the tumour and the normal area, respectively, for real-time monitoring. The tumour was cooled to an internal temperature of $-20°C$, after which a nephrostomy tube was placed inside the tumour.

After percutaneous cryosurgery, the kidney on the affected side, including the tumour, was necrotic and shrunken (Fig. 22.5). The reduction rate in patient 1 was 68% 1 month after the procedure and 81%, 8 months later; that in patient 2 was 20% 1 month later. The size of the tumour in patient 3 was not stable 1 month later. The dyspnoea in patient 1 gradually improved and the chest radiograph was stable. The bone pain in patient 2 gradually disappeared in spite of there being no change in the bone metastasis. The severe cough in patient 3 improved and the chest radiograph was stable 1 month later. Both patients 1 and 2 became temporarily active 3 months later and the third patient 1 month later. They were followed up as outpatients. The Karnofsky performance scales in patients 1 and 2, 3 months after the procedure, rose to 60 and 70%, respectively, and that in patient 3, 1 month later, to 70%. Patient 1 died from cachexia 10 months postoperatively. The pelvic bone metastasis in patient 2 gradually increased from 4 months postoperatively and he died from dyspnoea 1 month later. Although the general condition of patient 3 is not vigorous, he is still alive with a performance scale of 70% at the time of reporting (Table 22.1).

Discussion

Since the development of an apparatus using liquid nitrogen, cryosurgery has been propagated for the treatment of superficial diseases in the fields of dermatology, gynaecology and otorhinolaryngology.[1,2] For deep lesions such as hepatoma it has been used only by direct exposure on open surgery.[3]

In urology, Gonder and his colleagues[4] reported an experimental study for the application of cryosurgery to prostatic disease in 1964. Transurethral cryotherapy for prostatic diseases has been widely performed since that report. However, the procedure involved some complications, such as urinary tract infections, delayed separation of necrotic material with

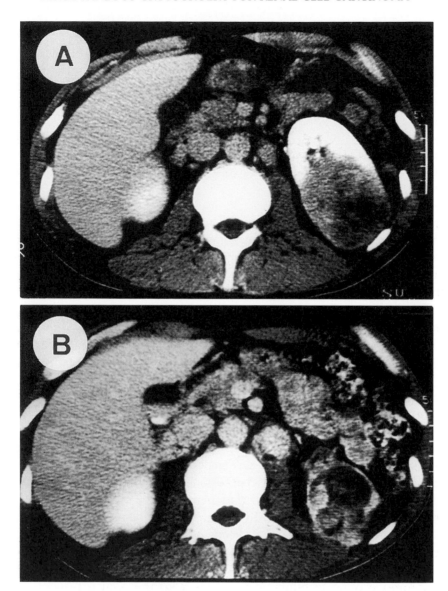

Fig. 22.5. Computerized tomography (CT) scan, patient 1: (A) CT shows left advanced renal cell carcinoma with swelling of para-aortic lymph nodes; (B) CT film 8 months after percutaneous cryosurgery shows that the affected kidney became necrotic and shrunken.

subsequent urinary tract obstruction, and cold injury to the bladder, ureters and rectum. Flocks and his colleagues[5] developed cryosurgery by the open perineal approach in 1972. Bonney and his colleagues[6] reported in 1982 that the long-term survival data for open perineal cryosurgery in prostastic cancer was equal to that of radical prostatectomy and radiation therapy.

Recently, the percutaneous technique with interventional ultrasound has made rapid progress in urology, contributing to renal biopsy[7] and

Patient		RR* (postop) (%)		KPS†(%)		Status (postop)
No.	Age (years)			Before	Postop	
1	48	81	(8)‡	10	60 (3)	Dead (10)
2	65	20	(1)	40	70 (3)	Dead (5)
3	62	Stable (1)		60	70 (1)	Alive (2)

Table 22.1. Results of percutaneous cryosurgery

*RR, reduction rate; †KPS, Karnofsky performance scales; ‡time of postoperative assessment (months) in parentheses.

endoscopic surgery such as percutaneous nephroureterolithotomy.[8] Even a target 1 cm in diameter can be penetrated accurately by this technique. Onik and his colleagues[9] introduced the technique to transperineal cryosurgery for prostatic cancer in 1991 and percutaneous prostatic cryosurgery is gaining widespread acceptance at present.

The modality for advanced renal cell carcinoma, especially with macrohaematuria, is mainly by open surgery, because the effective rates are not high although chemotherapy, the administration of interferon and embolization of the renal artery have become established. It was considered to be important to study the feasibility of percutaneous cryosurgery as a new method of management of advanced renal cell carcinoma. Renal puncture is thought to have caused the dissemination of the cancer cells. However, the authors believe that the risk of seeding cancer cells is no greater for the kidney than for other organs, because Abe and Saitoh[10] reported that no seeding in 36 renal tumour biopsies has been encountered during follow-ups ranging from 1 to 7 years, except for one case of angiomyoliposarcoma. The fundamental results showed that percutaneous cryosurgery could be effectively used in the treatment of renal cell carcinoma.

Percutaneous cryosurgery has been performed successfully in three patients with hypervascular renal tumours. No complications were encountered in this series. The monitoring of cryosurgery is clinically important in order to minimize the damage to the normal tissues. Two thermometers 0.5 mm in diameter and 25 cm in length were placed 1 cm from the cryoprobe and at the edge of the tumour. During cryosurgery, the degree of cooling was kept stable at $-20°C$ by monitoring the thermometers and the cooling process was observed by real-time ultrasound. After cryosurgery, the kidneys in patients 1 and 2 became necrotic and shrunken, including the tumour. The tumour in patient 3, originating in the ventral side of the kidney, became partially necrotic and the size of the kidney, including the tumour, was stable. Cryosurgery could not be performed in a manner that precluded side effects to the alimentary organs. After cryosurgery, no macrohaematuria occurred in patients 1 and

2. The Karnofsky performance scale in patients 1 and 2 showed a marked improvement 3 months after the operation but their general condition then deteriorated. That in patient 3 showed a slight improvement 1 month after the procedure and his general condition was stable. An immunological effect of cryosurgery could be presumed in assessing the mechanism of the temporary improvement.

These clinical results have demonstrated the following advantages of percutaneous cryosurgery for advanced renal cell carcinoma: (1) the procedure is available for the management of macrohaematuria because the affected kidney, including the tumour, becomes necrotic and shrunken; (2) the procedure can be performed without any complications; (3) the patient shows a temporary improvement in performance after the procedure.

Further studies will be required to assess whether the procedure is effective in early stage cases.

Acknowledgements

We thank Dr J. Y. Kuo for supplying us with renal cell cancer cell lines (NC-65).

This work was supported by a Grant-in-Aid for Scientific Research (C) from the Ministry of Education, Science and Culture, Japan.

References

1. Cooper I S, Lee A S J. Cryothalamectomy—hypothermic congelation. A technical advance in basal ganglia surgery. Preliminary report. J Am Geriatr Soc 1961; 9: 714–718
2. Cahan W G. Cryosurgery: the management of massive recurrent cancer. In: Leden H, Cahan W G (eds) Cryogenics in surgery. Tokyo: Medical Examination Publishing/Igaku-Shoin, 1971: 191
3. Ravikumar T S, Steele G D J. Hepatic cryosurgery. Surg Clin North Am 1989; 69: 433–440
4. Gonder M J, Soanes W A, Smith V. Experimental prostate cryosurgery. Invest Urol 1964; 1: 610–619
5. Flocks R H, Nelson C M K, Boatman D L. Perineal cryosurgery for prostatic carcinoma. J Urol 1972; 108: 933–935
6. Bonney W W, Fallon B, Gerber W L et al. Cryosurgery in prostatic cancer: survival. Urology 1982; 19: 37–42
7. Saitoh M. Selective renal biopsy under ultrasonic real-time guidance. Urol Radiol 1984; 6: 30–37
8. Saitoh M, Uchida M, Hashimoto T et al. Percutaneous nephroureterolithotomy. Review of 531 cases and a description of a new procedure. Jpn J Endourol ESWL 1988; 1: 22–25
9. Onik G, Porterfield B, Rubinsky B, Cohen J. Percutaneous transperineal prostate cryosurgery using transrectal ultrasound guidance: animal model. Urology 1991; 37: 277–281
10. Abe M, Saitoh M. Selective renal tumour biopsy under ultrasonic guidance. Br J Urol 1992; 70: 7–11

Use of lasers and cryotherapy for tumour destruction   *23*

A. C. von Eschenbach

Introduction

Each year approximately 20–25% of all newly diagnosed malignancies involve the genitourinary system. In order to treat these diseases effectively, especially in their early stages, urological surgeons are constantly seeking new and more effective methods of tumour destruction. This impetus, combined with our inherent fascination with instruments and devices, has resulted in urology being at the forefront of the development of new medical technology. Urologists are often among the first to apply new diagnostic or therapeutic modalities. These new ventures are usually initially associated with great excitement and enthusiasm, especially on the part of the investigators and those with a vested interest in the technology. However, in many cases the promise of great progress is not rapidly fulfilled and this early fascination gives way to disappointment and disillusionment, with many abandoning the effort. Unfortunately, too often in such a scenario, although the great potential benefits are still possible, promise gives way to problems before that potential is realized. This is a complex dilemma with its roots in unbridled enthusiasm, economic opportunities and insufficient education. In the rush to bring new technology from the laboratory to the bedside, important key prerequisites are ignored. Before any claim of efficacy or benefit can be made, arduous and meticulous, well-designed and well-conducted laboratory and clinical trials must be performed and critically assessed. Short cuts and premature pronouncements, no matter how well intentioned, will do more to retard progress than facilitate it. The story of the introduction of lasers and the recent resurgence of interest in cryoablation underscores many of these issues.

The availability of lasers for treating urological cancers in the 1980s was met with enthusiasm and dedication. These instruments seemed almost magical in their effects. Many surgeons bought expensive equipment requiring costly education of personnel, and patients were recruited for therapy that the surgeons expected to have wonderful effects. Today in many centres, this enthusiasm has now given way to disappointment and lack of interest. The equipment is infrequently used, for relatively few indications. This is regrettable because the potential for major progress remains.

Within the past few years the use of cryoablation, an old and established method of tumour destruction, has undergone a resurgence of interest. It was previously used (although subsequently abandoned) for treatment of prostate cancer; its resurgence is due to the availability of sophisticated ultrasound imaging, and new elegant technology that permits the percutaneous placement of multiple small-diameter probes within the prostate. Premature enthusiasm is already vying with unwarranted scepticism to obscure the scientific and clinical questions of whether this new technology has merit. The merits of new technology, its proper application and its shortcomings must all be defined by carefully conducted research in the laboratory and in the clinic, so that the lessons thus learned may lead to the development of even better technology. This chapter attempts to analyse critically the progress that has been made and the lessons learned from the experience of laser treatment of urological cancer and cryoablation of prostate cancer.

Use of lasers for genitourinary cancers

The distinctive properties of this unique form of energy have resulted in an almost unlimited repertoire of applications for military weapons, industry, telecommunications and medicine.

The medical applications of laser energy have often been developed empirically rather than designed for specific needs. The lasers currently available can have a variety of effects on tissue, as depicted in Fig. 23.1. Of these effects, the two that have been most exploited for tumour destruction are the photothermal and photochemical effects.

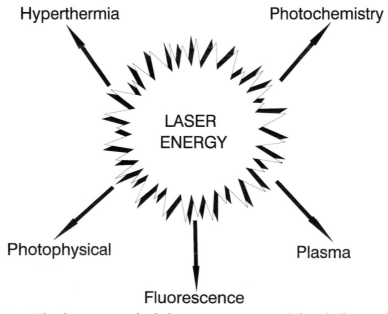

Fig. 23.1. *When laser energy is absorbed, it can cause a variety of physical effects in cells and tissues depending upon the wavelength, the power and duration of exposure.*

Photothermal tumour destruction

When laser electromagnetic energy of various wavelengths is applied to tissue, it is differentially absorbed by various cellular constituents and converted to another form of energy. This phenomenon accounts for the wide variety of lasers. In the infrared region of the electromagnetic spectrum, absorption is primarily by cell water and energy is converted to heat. At the far end of the region, the carbon dioxide (CO_2) laser, with a wavelength of 10060 nm, is very avidly absorbed by cell water; energy conversion to heat therefore takes place completely and instantaneously upon contact, resulting in a very rapid rise to extreme temperatures, with carbonization and vaporization of tissue. In the near-infrared region, the neodymium:yttrium aluminium garnet (Nd:YAG) laser, with a wavelength of 1060 nm, has a lower coefficient of absorption by water and this permits the light energy to penetrate and disperse deeper into tissues with a more gradual build-up of heat and a more gradual rise in temperature. The contrast between these two laser effects is akin to the difference between broiling and baking. The vaporization power of the CO_2 laser makes it an ideal tool for cutting and ablating tissue, whereas the Nd:YAG wavelength permits transmission by way of thin flexible optical fibres and through a fluid medium, and is ideal for coagulation of tissue. Although the CO_2 laser had been used by a variety of specialities, such as gynaecology, it was the introduction of the Nd:YAG laser that popularized the use of lasers in urology. Hoffstetter and others[1-3] must take the credit for their pioneering effort in developing the clinical applications of the Nd:YAG laser, especially for the endoscopic destruction of bladder and upper tract tumours, and for lesions of the external genitalia. Following reports that tumours could be as effectively destroyed with such lasers as with the use of standard therapy such as electrocoagulation, and with excellent cosmetic and functional results, urologists enthusiastically embraced this new technology. However, some shortcomings were apparent.

Although the physics of laser energy generation are very precise, the biology of its effects on tissues is empirical. Parameters of ideal power, time and area of irradiation could not be transferred easily from the laboratory to the operating room. The interaction of laser energy and biological tissue is a complex process; it is affected by chromophores in cells, such as haemoglobin, myoglobin or melanin, and changes as the lasing process changes the optical properties of the tissues. The best estimate of the effects in tissue were the visible changes occurring on the surface of the tissue. The answer to clinicians who asked 'How much and for how long do I laser bladder tumours?' was 'Until they turn white' (Fig. 23.2). Furthermore, it was thought that laser destruction would result in a lower incidence of recurrence of bladder tumours, but experience has confirmed that most tumour recurrences are a function of the biology of bladder cancer rather than of the modality employed for the primary tumour.

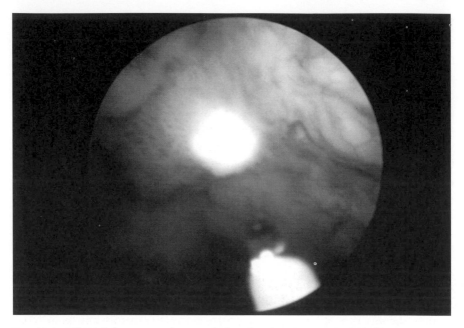

Fig. 23.2. Nd:YAG laser energy being applied to the edge of a superficial bladder tumour until coagulation is achieved and the tissue becomes white.

The initial enthusiasm and excitement over this new, wonderful tool gave way to uncertainty regarding its value and appropriate application in the treatment of bladder cancer. A prospective randomized trial by Beisland and Seland[4] helped to define some of these issues. For patients with stage T_1 and T_2 tumours, 62 were treated with the Nd:YAG laser and 60 by transurethral resection (TUR). Small tumours (<6 mm) did not recur in the treated area, regardless of the modality, suggesting that the laser and TUR were of equivalent efficacy. However, larger tumours were more likely to recur in the treated area when treated by TUR alone (19/44) compared with TUR followed by laser therapy (3/44). In untreated areas of the bladder, the frequency of recurrence was approximately 20% and was equivalent between the two groups, suggesting that out-of-field recurrences were not reduced by the use of the laser. The fact that laser irradiation does not alter the biology of bladder cancer and cannot be expected to influence disease outside the treated field has been documented by a number of investigators.[5]

In spite of its advantage in reducing in-field recurrences, the use of the laser as an adjunct to TUR has not gained widespread acceptance. In part, this is due to technical problems: for example, once an aggressive resection has been performed, there is a lack of precise endpoints for laser therapy. The application of sufficient energy is uncertain because the optical properties of tissue have been altered by the TUR and the operator has no means of estimating subsurface coagulating effects. The presence or absence of blood or char, and the depth of the resection, will significantly influence the absorption and transmission of laser energy. This lack of precision is even more problematic if tumours are thought to be muscle invasive. A number of studies (Table 23.1) have confirmed that as tumours increase in stage, there is a much greater likelihood of failure of laser irradiation to eradicate disease. Tarantino et al[6] treated 18 patients with bladder cancer prior to radical cystectomy: of 12 patients with stage T_2, only two had no evidence of tumour in the cystectomy specimen (T_0) whereas ten patients had a tumour of higher stage. These authors pointed out the problems of lack of accurate staging of the bladder tumour and of certifying that the extent of coagulation is adequate for complete tumour destruction deep in the bladder wall.

Combining laser irradiation with TUR is cumbersome and time-consuming for the surgeon, and the results for large and potentially invasive tumours are not sufficiently compelling to support its routine use. The role of lasers for thermal destruction of bladder tumours remains limited until problems of predicting and monitoring subsurface effects are resolved. Other advances such as contact tips, alternative wavelengths such as the argon, potassium titanyl phosphate (KTP) and holmium:YAG (Ho:YAG) lasers have not improved upon the results achieved with the Nd:YAG, nor have they provided any resolution to the problem of subsurface dosimetry.

Ureteral and pelvic tumours

The laser is perhaps the ideal method of destroying tumours of the ureter and renal pelvis. The latest flexible, small-calibre (yet steerable) pyeloureteroscopes provide excellent visualization of the collecting

Authors	Patients (n)	Response
Shanberg et al[17]	53	T_1, 18% recurrence; T_2, 33% recurrence; T_3, 80% recurrence
McPhee et al[18]	32	T_2, 12/12 NED* at 6–78 months; T_3, 8/14 persistent; T_4, 6/6 persistent
Smith[19]		T_2, 82% NED at 6 month follow-up; T_{3a}, 54% NED at 6 month follow-up; T_{3b}, 32% NED at 6 month follow-up
Beisland and Sander[20]	15	T_2, ten alive NED, one dead NED, four recurrences requiring cystectomy

Table 23.1. Results of laser therapy in invasive bladder cancer
*NED, no evidence of disease.

system. Quartz fibres are available that have a diameter of 200–400 μm and that can pass easily along the operating channel of these instruments, to be aimed at the tumour visualized. An attempt is made to deliver laser radiation at right angles to the tumour, and it is desirable to have contact and optical fibres with an angled tip to deliver the energy obliquely.

In a review of endoscopic management of upper tract tumours, Gerber and Lyon point out that advances in endourological techniques have made successful treatment of tumours in the upper tract quite feasible, especially when employing the Nd:YAG laser.[7] This fact has been substantiated by a number of investigators (Table 23.2). Despite its effectiveness, however, there are limitations to this approach and cases must be carefully selected. Small tumours in the ureter are easier to visualize and treat. In the renal pelvis and calyceal collecting system, access to tumours can be quite difficult and frustrating. Inspection is usually satisfactory, but when the laser fibre is inserted in the working channel, the range of deflection of the scope and the flow of irrigating fluid are both impaired, impeding treatment. For many renal pelvic tumours, a percutaneous approach via a nephrostomy placed through a portion of the kidney that affords direct access to the lesion is preferable. With this approach, rather than a ureteroscope, a flexible nephroscope with a larger-diameter operating channel can be used. Similarly, rigid endoscopes are quite difficult to employ for renal pelvic and calyceal tumours, but they can be ideal for ureteral lesions. When laser energy is applied appropriately, upper tract tumours can be effectively destroyed without risk of perforation or bleeding. As with bladder tumours, the utilization of this technique is limited by the lack of control of the depth of irradiation, and the uncertainty that all of the cancer has been destroyed. It is crucial, therefore, to include only those patients with small,

Authors	Patients (n)	Response
Schilling et al[21]	16 Ureter	Two strictures; no local tumour recurrences (follow-up 3–31 months)
Blute et al[22]	11	Two recurrences at 9 and 23 months; in all, NED* with 2nd treatment
Carson[23]	8	In all, NED at 6–40 months
Grossman et al[24]	8 Pelvis/ureter	26 treatments; two patient failures
Johnson[25]	3 Ureter	In all, NED at 5, 7 and 22 months; no stricture; one extravasation
Gaboardi et al[26]	18	In ten, NED at 6–30 months (one nephrectomy)

Table 23.2. Results of laser therapy for tumours in the renal pelvis and ureter
*NED, no evidence of disease.

low-grade tumours and in whom conservative management is justified and the probability of success is quite high.

Prostate cancer

Successful endoscopic thermal laser destruction of urothelial cancers has stimulated interest in adaptation of this technology for the treatment of tumours of the prostate. Because prostate cancers are peripheral in location, the most feasible application was a technique of TUR of the central prostate followed by Nd:YAG irradiation of the prostatic fossa. By directing the laser through both a transurethral and suprapubic cystostomy approach, the entire prostate bed, including the base and the apex of the gland, could be uniformly irradiated. With more than 60 months' follow-up, Beisland and Sander[8] reported on 110 of 124 patients who were without evidence of disease for as long as 114 months, and the actuarial disease-free survival was 88% at 4–9 years. Only six patients had local recurrence, three of whom were treated early in the series before using the suprapubic approach. Severe incontinence was reported in only one patient.

Because the Nd:YAG wavelength penetrates the prostatic tissue to a depth of approximately 5–7 mm, it facilitates the effective eradication of tumour in the periphery of the prostate; however, there is no means of accurately assessing the extent of thermal destruction. Following TUR, the varying optical properties of the surface being irradiated can make a dramatic difference to energy absorption. To avoid such problems, a period of at least 4 weeks should be left until all blood clot and eschar has resolved. In addition, the thickness of the peripheral zone may be quite variable and McNicholas and colleagues[9] have pointed out the necessity of performing an 'extended' TUR, in order to make the peripheral zone as thin as possible, and of evaluating the extent of resection by the use of transrectal ultrasound to measure thickness, because of the often surprising underestimation of the amount of residual tissue present. The more aggressive prostatic resection increases the possibility of complications, especially bleeding. Of 17 patients with a mean follow-up of 6 months (range 1–14 months) two with excessive residual tissue had positive biopsies initially and were rendered disease free after a second treatment. Two patients continue to have persistently positive biopsies, but biopsies are negative in the remainder. Using a similar technique, Samdal and Brevik[10] reported on 26 men with a follow-up of 6–42 months (mean 21 months); 22 patients are reported as free of disease. Only three patients had prostate needle biopsies and all were negative for tumour. Late complications occurred in eight patients; these complications included a bladder neck contracture in four and severe stress incontinence in two patients.

As prostate cancers often have unrecognized microscopic extensions beyond the prostatic border, it is desirable to photoirradiate slightly beyond the margins of the prostate. This necessitates using some method of ensuring that normal tissues are not damaged. One suggestion has been to place a finger with a thermocouple on its tip into the rectum to monitor the temperature of the rectal wall and to cease irradiation before the temperature is greater than 45°C. Obviously, the difference between safe irradiation for the rectum and effective irradiation for the prostate cancer can often be very small. Despite the technical challenges, preliminary results attest to the promise of thermal destruction of prostate cancer. However, these current methods of photoirradiating the prostate are cumbersome and have not provided sufficient advantages over conventional therapy to promote widespread use. There are, however, many possibilities for major improvements. Instead of topical irradiation of the prostatic bed, it would be ideal to use interstitial fibres for delivery of irradiation to the entire gland, thereby enhancing treatment of the periphery and obviating the need for TUR. Interstitial fibres have been applied to the treatment of benign prostatic hyperplasia and can be placed under ultrasound guidance into the peripheral portion of the gland. In the future, these interstitial fibres could be linked to diode lasers that are ideally suited for slow, low-power irradiation which would facilitate wide dispersion of heat. Feedback systems are needed that could modulate the laser power, and ultrasound may be adapted to monitor temperature rise within and around the prostate to give an indication of the optimal dose of energy. There is also great potential to enhance tumour cell destruction by combining the hyperthermic effects of the laser with photodynamic therapy, using the same interstitial fibre for delivery of both laser energies.

External genitalia

Thus far, perhaps the greatest contribution of laser technology to clinical urology is the ability to destroy superficial lesions of the external genitalia with excellent cosmetic and functional preservation. The laser, particularly the Nd:YAG, has become the treatment of choice for extensive condyloma acuminata and low-stage penile carcinoma. The Nd:YAG is usually preferred because it affords coagulation of the lesion and any microscopic subsurface extension. The CO_2 laser is also used, but is best chosen when superficial vaporization of a genital lesion is desired, such as for the treatment of balanitis xerotica obliterans.

Although there are other effective therapies for superficial penile cancer, such as Moh's surgery, radiation therapy and topical chemotherapy, the laser is the most desirable. For lesions of comparable size, the laser most reliably achieves immediate tumour destruction with the least mutilating effect on the appearance and function of the penis. A number of studies with long-term follow-up have confirmed the efficacy of this procedure for tumours that are small and only superficially invasive (Table 23.3). For large

Authors	Patients (n)	Response
Rothenberger[27]	17	No recurrences; mean follow-up 5 years
Bandieramonte et al[28]	10	One recurrence at 4 months
Malloy et al[29]	16	T_{IS}, 5/5 NED* at 12–36 months follow-up; T_1, 6/9 NED at 12–36 months follow-up; T_2, 0/2 NED at 12–36 months follow-up
Boon[30]	16	Three recurrences; mean follow-up 17 months
von Eschenbach et al[31]	10	Two recurrences at 7 and 15 months; all NED with 2nd treatment; mean follow-up 32 months
Horenblas et al[32]	17	3 (18%) local recurrences

Table 23.3. Results of laser therapy in penile cancer
*NED, no evidence of disease.

and deeply invasive lesions, penile amputation continues to be mandatory. Technical developments that have been employed to enhance the results of laser therapy include the use of contact tips for surface denudation of carcinoma in situ and the exploration of alternative wavelengths of energy, including the KTP, Ho:YAG and argon lasers. These tools offer some variation with regard to tissue absorption, but have not substantially expanded the repertoire. Given the problems posed by deeply invasive or extensive tumours, it is not likely that any developments in future laser technology will significantly improve on the current results achieved by Nd:YAG irradiation.

Photochemical applications

Photodynamic therapy represents the most promising future application of lasers in the field of oncology. The concept of the selective photoactivation of a lethal drug present in a cancer cell, without affecting nearby normal cells, is intriguing. Because of its power and selectivity with regard to wavelengths, the laser is an ideal source of light for photoactivation. The photoactivation of a compound kills principally by the intracellular production of singlet oxygen, which reacts to produce free radicals or peroxides that damage cellular constituents such as DNA and mitochondria.

It is now apparent that the effects of photodynamic therapy may involve further damage by at least two other mechanisms. The endothelial cells of the microvasculature supplying the tumour may be particularly susceptible to damage because of a higher drug concentration around blood vessels. This causes disruption of the blood vessels with subsequent thrombosis and haemorrhage. Furthermore, these damaged endothelial cells can release powerful cytokines such as interleukins and tumour necrosis factor (TNF) that can mediate cytotoxicity of the neighbouring tumour cells. These varied mechanisms of tumour cell destruction are only now being appreciated and studied. The use of laser photodynamic therapy has been advocated by Dougherty and Marcus,[11] who proposed the use of a derivative of haematoporphyrin (HPD) as a photosensitizing agent for the treatment of bladder cancer. The dye is photoactivated by interacting with light of a specific wavelength. The ideal absorption wavelength for HPD photoactivation is actually in the green–blue range of the spectrum, but because tissue penetration of light is greater at longer wavelengths, 630 nm was chosen in the red portion of the spectrum so that photoactivation would occur deeper within the tissues. An argon laser was used as an energy source to excite the red dye rhodamine B, which then emitted laser energy at the desired wavelength. This laser light could then be transmitted by optical quartz fibres through the endoscope into the bladder. The light could be shone on a discrete area, or the whole bladder wall could be illuminated. From the outset of photodynamic therapy, a number of problems have existed: for example, the optimal dose of photosensitizer must be established; the dose and the timing of applications of laser energy may not be optimal; the use of a dye laser pumped by another laser is expensive and cumbersome, and demands a high degree of technical skill for its operation; achieving a uniform distribution of light energy throughout the entire volume of tumour and over the entire surface of the bladder remains quite a challenge, despite many ingenious devices intended to achieve uniform dosimetry.

Although initial clinical trials were fairly promising, with claims by a number of investigators of complete tumour destruction of superficial carcinoma in situ in over 70% of patients (Table 23.4), papillary tumours or

Author	No. of tumours	Response*			Relapse	Follow-up (months)
		CR	PR	NR		
Benson[33]	15 focal	15	0	0	8	6–32
	12 diffuse	12	0	0	2	Mean: 7
Nseyo et al[34]	6	3	2	1	—	2 to > 12
Harty et al[35]	2	1	0	1	0	—
Prout et al[36]	3	3	0	0	3	—
Total	38	34	2	2		

Table 23.4. Photodynamic therapy in bladder cancer: carcinoma in situ (T_{IS})
*CR, complete response; PR, partial response; NR, no response.

Authors	No. and stage of tumours	Response*			Follow-up (months)
		CR	PR	NR	
Benson[33]	2 T_a	0	0	2	—
Shumaker and Hetzel[37]	4 T_a	2	0	2	6–15
Nseyo et al[34]	8 T_a	3	3	2	2 to > 12
	8 T_1	2	5	1	
Prout et al[36]	50 T_a/T_1	12	25	13	3
Harty et al[35]	3 T_a	3	0	0	—
	2 T_1	1	0	1	—
Total	77	23	33	21	

Table 23.5. Photodynamic therapy in superficial papillary T_a/T_1 bladder cancer

*CR, complete response; PR, partial response; NR, no response.

invasive tumours did not seem to respond (Table 23.5). Furthermore, patients usually encountered severe and prolonged irritative urinary symptoms of frequency, urgency and dysuria, and some patients eventually developed debilitating contracted bladders. As a haematoporphyrin is absorbed and retained in the skin, cutaneous photosensitization occurs and can last for as long as 4–6 weeks, during which patients cannot be exposed to sunlight or intense artificial light. These problems were substantial, and caused many to be reluctant to embrace this new therapy. Despite problems with this specific application of drug and device, the potential of photodynamic therapy for selective tumour cell destruction demands that research into new drugs, laser systems and delivery modes should continue.

New agents that are of interest include 5-aminolevulinic acid (5-ALA)—which can be administered orally, is endogenously activated to protoporphyrin IX and accumulates in mucosal tissues—and a variety of photosensitizing compounds such as the chlorins, phthalocyanines, benzoporphyrin and doxycyclin. New drug delivery systems, such as liposome encapsulation, can be further explored. Transillumination by interstitially placed fibres is particularly attractive for treating solid tumours.

Beyond bladder cancer, photodynamic therapy has exceptional opportunities for the treatment of prostate cancer and renal cell carcinoma. Of particular interest is the potential for transperineal percutaneous photoirradiation of the prostate.

The lack of progress of photodynamic therapy is not because the concept is flawed, but because research has not yet produced the ideal combination of laser energy and drugs. The development of clinically effective photosensitizing drugs cannot stop with HPD, any more than the development of antibiotics should have stopped after penicillin or antimetabolites after nitrogen mustard. Further research is needed to exploit the molecular and cellular mechanisms of damage after photodynamic therapy. There is yet much potential for progress, despite the problems that have been encountered.

Other laser effects

Beyond the thermal and photodynamic effects of laser energy, tumour cells may be affected by lasers in a variety of other ways. Laser absorption by organic cellular constituents can produce physical shock waves that can damage or alter delicate cell structures. Some wavelengths of light energy have direct biological effects on cells, as evidenced by ultraviolet light stimulating the production of melanin and vitamin D. It is conceivable that direct cellular, physical and biochemical effects, as yet undiscovered, may be modulated by laser energy. A whole new field of photobiology must be explored as a foundation for such new, potentially wondrous applications.

The initial promises offered for the laser may have been premature and, perhaps appropriately, were soon curtailed by a recognition of the problems, pitfalls and limitations of currently available technology; however, the potential is real and clinical and laboratory researchers may yet expand the healing power of this wonderful form of energy.

Cryotherapy

In clinical medicine and in the research laboratory, cold is used most often to preserve cells and tissues; however, freezing is also an old and well-established method of destruction. Much more is known about the optimal conditions for cryopreservation, but rapidly freezing to very low temperatures, which produces intracellular ice, followed by a slow thaw is a very effective method of cell destruction.

When technology became available by which liquid nitrogen could be circulated through metal probes to produce extremely cold temperatures at their tips, cryoablation became an additional weapon for urologists to use to destroy tumours. Specially designed probes could be inserted into the urethra that allowed the freezing tip to be positioned at the level of the prostate.[12] An alternative approach was to expose the prostate via a perineal surgical incision and to place the probe tip directly on the posterior surface of the prostate.[13]

Freezing by these methods proved to be quite effective for the destruction of prostatic tissue and the survival of patients treated with cryoablation alone or cryoablation plus hormonal therapy was comparable to that seen for other forms of therapy.[14] However, the extent of freezing within the tissue was uncertain, and areas of prostate cancer that were a considerable distance from the probe were likely to be undertreated. Similarly, the freezing process could extend indiscriminately to surrounding normal structures, such as the perineum, rectum and bladder neck, with troublesome complications. This technology was judged to be cumbersome, imprecise and, at times, associated with difficult complications; the use of cryotherapy for prostate cancer therefore gave way to advances being made in other modalities such as surgery, radiation therapy and androgen ablation.

However, within the past few years, the advent of sophisticated ultrasound technology, which makes possible the visualization of the internal architecture of the prostate with a high degree of resolution and clarity, has stimulated interest in ultrasound-guided percutaneous transperineal cryoablation of the prostate. Onik and Cohen[15] have developed a method for this procedure, using the new technology. The University of Texas M. D. Anderson Cancer Center's Department of Urology purchased the first Acuprobe® cryotherapy machine that became commercially available from Cryomedical Sciences, Rockville, MD, USA. Since July 1992, at this institution the system has been used in a phase I/II study to evaluate the safety and efficacy of this new method of cryoablation as salvage therapy for patients with biopsy-proven local recurrence of prostate cancer following definitive therapy. Until this study has been completed, the method has not been employed here as primary therapy; however, it has been used as primary therapy at other centres in the United States.

The technique of this method of cryoablation is quite elegant. Under direct ultrasound imaging, one to five probes are placed percutaneously into the prostate in a geometric configuration that will facilitate the complete and uniform freezing of a selected volume of prostate tissue, thereby directing the freezing process to any site of the prostate tumour, including areas of extraprostatic tumour extension. Most importantly, in addition to visualizing the precise localization of the probes, ultrasound also enables the operator to observe the development of the 'ice ball' of frozen tissue within the prostate. This imaging of the frozen zone is possible because, as tissue freezes, it becomes densely echogenic, resulting in the appearance of a very distinct white echogenic rim at the edge of the ice ball, beyond which is a black anechoic area due to through shadowing (Fig. 23.3). As no visualization is possible beyond the echogenic interface, the fate of structures beyond the interface cannot be directly observed, which is a potential shortcoming of this technique. However, in practice, the freezing process is begun with the anteriorly placed probes, and the ice ball can be allowed to migrate from anterior to posterior; with transrectal ultrasound monitoring, the migration of the freezing process towards the rectum can be halted before it extends through the muscularis propria of the rectal wall. The freezing is monitored in both axial and longitudinal planes, and the cephalad extension into the bladder base and seminal

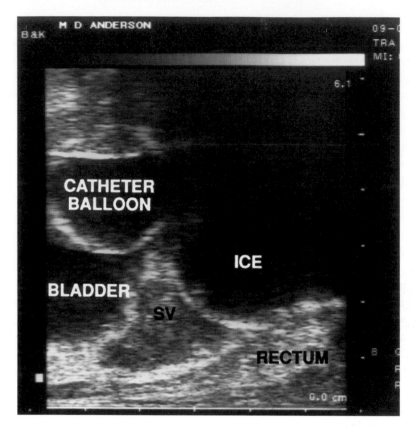

Fig. 23.3. *Longitudinal transrectal ultrasound view of the development of an ice ball within the prostate. The white echogenic rim of frozen tissue is quite distinctive. SV, seminal vesicle.*

vesicles and the caudad migration into the urogenital diaphragm can also be closely monitored.

This superb ability to localize and control the freezing process accurately makes modern cryoablation a vastly better procedure than it was 20–30 years ago. Preliminary analysis of 76 radiation-failure patients treated between July 1992 and March 1994 supports this contention. Among these patients, the procedure was quite safe and its effectiveness in tumour destruction was impressive. Of 51 patients who had postcryoablation biopsies 6 months after percutaneous cryoablation, 39 (76.5%) were biopsy negative for tumour. Among the 12 patients with a positive biopsy, six had only a microscopic focus of residual cancer involving less than 5% of the biopsy specimen. More recently, the author's team has modified the procedure, first to freeze completely, then to thaw completely and subsequently to refreeze again rapidly in the hope of improving tumour cell kill. In their initial experience with this technique, the negative biopsy rate is approximately 90%. The modern technology of a percutaneous approach used in this technique requires minimum hospitalization and allows a rapid return to full activity. Although no severe perioperative complications have occurred, most patients experience some degree of morbidity, usually involving rectal or perineal discomfort (especially when sitting), bladder irritability and temporary urinary obstruction. Only one patient developed a serious complication, with sepsis due to a prostatic abscess occurring approximately 2 weeks after therapy. Most troublesome has been the development of some degree of urinary incontinence in 46% of patients. This is usually in the form of mild stress incontinence that improves over time, but it has persisted for at least 6 months in 28% of patients thus far.

Other investigators have employed this form of cryotherapy as the primary treatment for organ-confined (T_1/T_2) prostate cancer, or for extracapsular extension (T_3). Data from these early efforts are now becoming available and suggest that cryotherapy can achieve destruction of tumour, as evidenced by a high percentage of negative biopsies at various times following therapy. Miller and Cohen[16] have reported that in 62 patients with clinical stage T_3 tumours, 49 (79%) were negative on biopsy at 6 months. Of the 13 patients with positive biopsies, 12 underwent a second cryoablation and nine were negative on subsequent biopsy. However, whether these negative biopsies represent permanent and complete eradication of all local disease is unknown. Although almost all patients experience a decline in prostate-specific antigen (PSA) level following therapy, only a portion achieve an undetectable level, and it is uncertain whether this decline will be sustained.

Much research is needed to define the optimal freezing process in the human prostate and to develop methods that will ensure that all cancer cells will be maximally affected, regardless of proximity to the urethra or major blood vessels. It is interesting to speculate whether temporarily interrupting blood flow through the dorsal vein complex or the neurovascular bundles would improve the effectiveness of freezing for extracapsular extension. Optimal freezing parameters, such as the double-freeze cycle, need to be investigated, and the use of an ultrasound with colour Doppler flow capability may identify the presence and magnitude of such blood flow and monitor its selective destruction or interruption by the first freeze in order to ensure the success of a second freeze. The development of warmers to protect normal structures in a highly selective fashion that does not also spare tumour foci is essential in an effort to reduce morbidity.

Carefully designed and conducted clinical trials are mandatory to define the potential of this form of tumour destruction. Despite the very elegant nature of modern cryotherapy technology, results thus far are empirical and progress has been by trial and error. Already it is apparent that protection of the continence mechanism is needed, especially for patients whose tissues have already been compromised by prior therapy, such as radiation. A system for insertion of thermocouples at strategic points in and around the prostate may assist in defining the endpoints of therapy, it may also be used during the freezing process to assist in adjusting the varying rates of freezing within the prostate to better confine the freezing zone to the tumour and to protect normal structures. The efficacy of tumour cell destruction may be further enhanced by combining freezing with other strategies such as chemotherapy. By administering a dose of a chemotherapeutic agent before freezing, the drug may be preferentially trapped within the tissue after freezing, owing to interruption in blood flow and subsequent impaired drug clearance. These opportunities must first be addressed in the laboratory and then applied in the clinic if a strong foundation is to be established for the future safe and effective application of cryoablation. Modest current success should only serve as a stimulus and justification for investing in the research further to expand the application and reduce the morbidity of cryoablation. It is conceivable that the foundation established in the treatment of prostate cancer will serve as a stepping-off point for the cryoablation of other tumours such as renal cell carcinomas and bladder cancer.

Conclusions

The history of advances in laser and cryotechnology has taught us that progress comes in phases. In the beginning, there is *promise*, but the promise of great benefit often gives way to the era of *problems* when the limitations and complications become painfully apparent. At this point, it is tempting to discard and denigrate; however, in experiencing problems, one is also given a perspective of the true *potential* of these new tools. It then becomes apparent that we have only begun the process of discovery, not completed it. To kill selectively those cancer cells hidden deep in organs such as the prostate, bladder or kidney, using the various properties of laser energy or by insult of freezing, challenges the imagination and invites investigation. In this era of exploitation of technology, there is no substitute for research. If urologists are to be at the forefront of innovation and discovery, rather than riding the ebb and flow of empiricism, investment is essential in the critical but open-minded laboratory and clinical investigation is required to bring these new forms of energy to their full potential as cancer destroyers.

References

1. Hofstetter A, Frank F. The neodymium:YAG laser in urology. Basel: Roche, 1980: 72.
2. Staehler G, Hofstetter A. Transurethral laser irradiation of urinary bladder tumors. Eur Urol 1979; 5: 64–69
3. Staehler G, Halldorsson T, Langerholc J et al. Endoscopic applications of the neodymium:YAG laser in urology: theory, results, dosimetry. Urol Res 1981; 9: 45–51

4. Beisland H O, Seland P. A prospective randomized study of neodymium:YAG laser irradiation versus TUR in the treatment of urinary bladder cancer. Scand J Urol Nephrol 1986; 20: 209–212

5. von Eschenbach A C. Superficial bladder cancer. In: Smith J A Jr (ed) Lasers in urologic surgery, 2nd ed. Chicago: Year Book Medical, 1989: 57–66

6. Tarantino A E, Aretz H T, Libertino J A et al. Is the neodymium:YAG laser effective therapy for invasive bladder cancer? Urology 1991; 38: 514–518

7. Gerber G S, Lyon E S. Endourological management of upper tract urothelial tumors: review article. J Urol 1993; 150: 2–7

8. Beisland H O, Sandor S. Localized prostate carcinoma treated with TUR and neodymium:YAG laser irradiation. Scand J Urol Nephrol 1991; 138(suppl): 117–119

9. McNicholas T A, Carter S, Wickham J E, O'Donoghue E P. YAG laser treatment of early carcinoma of the prostate. Br J Urol 1988; 61: 239–243

10. Samdal F, Brevik B. Laser combined with TURP in the treatment of localized prostatic cancer. Scand J Urol Nephrol 1990; 24: 175–177

11. Dougherty T J, Marcus S L. Photodynamic therapy: feature article. Eur J Cancer 1992; 28: 1734–1742

12. Gonder M J, Soanes W A, Shulman S. Cryosurgical treatment of the prostate. Invest Urol 1976; 3: 372–378

13. Flocks R H, Nelson C M K, Boatman D L. Perineal cryosurgery for prostatic carcinoma. J Urol 1972; 108: 933–935

14. Bonney W W, Fallon B, Gerber W L et al. Cryosurgery in prostatic cancer: survival. Urology 1982; 14: 37–42

15. Onik G M, Cohen J K, Reyes G D et al. Transrectal ultrasound-guided percutaneous radical cryosurgical ablation of the prostate. Cancer 1993; 72: 1291–1299

16. Miller R J Jr, Cohen J K, Merlotti L A. Percutaneous transperineal cryosurgical ablation of the prostate for the primary treatment of clinical stage C adenocarcinoma of the prostate. Urology 1994; 44: 170–174

17. Shanberg A M, Chalfin S A, Tansey L A. Neodymium:YAG laser: new treatment for urethral stricture disease. Urology 1984; 24: 15–17

18. McPhee M S, Arnfield M R, Tulip J, Lakey W H. Neodymium:YAG laser therapy for infiltrating bladder cancer. J Urol 1988; 140: 44–46

19. Smith JA Jr. Invasive bladder cancer. In: Smith J A Jr (ed) Lasers in urologic surgery, 2nd ed. Chicago: Year Book Medical, 1989: 73–80

20. Beisland H O, Sander S. Neodymium:YAG laser irradiation of Stage T2 muscle invasive bladder cancer: long-term results. Br J Urol 1990; 65: 24–26

21. Schilling A, Bowering R, Keiditsch E. Use of Nd:YAG laser in treatment of ureteral tumors and ureteral condylomata acuminata. Eur Urol 1986; 12: 30–33

22. Blute M L, Segura J W, Patterson D E et al. Impact of endourology on diagnosis and management of upper urinary tract urothelial cancer. J Urol 1989; 141: 1298–1301

23. Carson C C, III. Endoscopic treatment of upper and lower urinary tract lesions using lasers. Semin Urol 1991; 9: 185

24. Grossman H B, Schwartz S L, Konnak J W. Ureteroscopic treatment of urothelial carcinoma of the ureter and renal pelvis. J Urol 1992; 148: 275–277

25. Johnson D E. Treatment of distal ureteral tumors using endoscopic argon photoirradiation. Lasers Surg Med 1992; 12: 490–493

26. Gaboardi F, Bozzola F, Dotti E, Galli L. Conservative treatment of upper urinary tract tumors with Nd:YAG laser. J Endourol 1994; 8: 37–41

27. Rothenberger K H. Value of the neodymium:YAG laser in the therapy of penile carcinoma. Eur Urol 1986; 12: 34–36

28. Bandieramonte G, Santoro O, Boracehi P et al. Total resection of the glans penis surface by CO_2 laser microsurgery. Acta Oncol 1988; 27: 575–578

29. Malloy T R, Wein A J, Carpiniello V L. Carcinoma of the penis treated with neodymium:YAG laser. Urology 1988; 31: 26–29

30. Boon T A. Sapphire probe laser surgery for localized carcinoma of the penis. Eur J Surg Oncol 1988; 14: 193–195

31. von Eschenbach A C, Johnson D E, Wishnow K I et al. Results of laser therapy for carcinoma of the penis: organ preservation. In: Smith P H, Pavone-Macaluso M (eds)

Urological oncology: reconstructive surgery, organ conservation and restoration of function. EORTC Genitourinary Group Monograph 10. New York: Wiley-Liss, 1991; 407–412

32. Horenblas S, van Tinteren H, Delemarre J F M et al. Squamous cell carcinoma of the penis II: treatment of the primary tumor. J Urol 1992; 147: 1533–1538

33. Benson R C Jr. Treatment of diffuse transitional cell carcinoma in situ by whole bladder hematoporphyrin derivative photodynamic therapy. J Urol 1985; 134: 675–678

34. Nseyo U O, Dougherty T J, Sullivan L. Photodynamic therapy in the management of resistant lower urinary tract carcinoma. Cancer 1987; 60: 3113–3119

35. Harty J I, Amin M, Wieman T J et al. Complications of whole bladder dihematoporphyrin ether photodynamic therapy. J Urol 1989; 141: 1341–1346

36. Prout G R, Lin C W, Benson R et al. Photodynamic therapy with hematoporphyrin derivative in the treatment of superficial transitional cell carcinoma of the bladder. N Engl J Med 1987; 317: 1251–1255

37. Shumaker B P, Hetzel F W. Clinical laser photodynamic therapy in the treatment of bladder carcinoma. Photochem Photobiol 1987; 46: 899–901

Index

INDEX